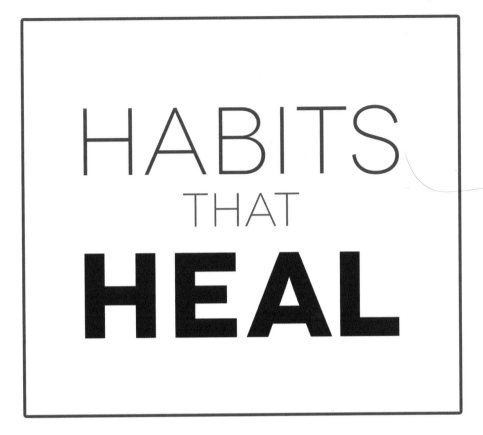

HABITS
THAT
HEAL

Habits from America's Longest Living People

Monica Fukuda with David K. Fukuda, M.D.

Unless otherwise indicated, all Scripture references are from the King James Version.

Scripture quotations marked NKJV are taken from the New King James Version.

Scripture quotations marked ESV are taken from the English Standard Version.

Scripture quotations marked A.R.V. are taken from the American Revised Version.

CAUTION:
The information in this book is not intended to replace medical advice or treatment. The reader should consult a medical professional in matters relating to his/her health and particularly with respect to any symptoms that may require diagnosis or medical attention.

Designed by Ricardo Camacho & Kayla Marcoux.
Cover Design by Robert Koorenny
The typefaces used are PT Sans and Lato.
Images: photodune.net, Ricardo Camacho, Brielle Anderson, Germain Rodriguez

ISBN: 978-0-9963380-0-4

CONTENTS

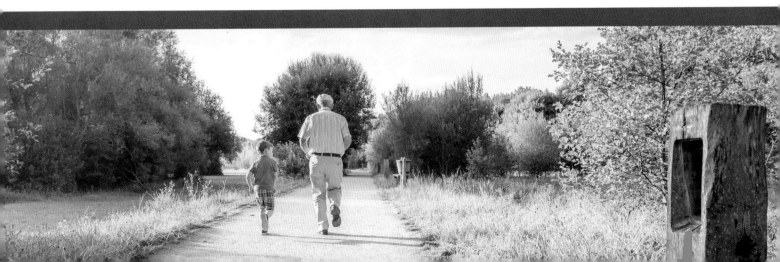

HOW TO USE THIS BOOK

WHY WAS THIS BOOK WRITTEN?

Well, in short, we want to change the world. We see so much disease, pain, and suffering in the precious lives around us, and we want to help alleviate that. We want to tell as many people as possible that there is another way. Our desire is to share with the world how true joy and peace, health and happiness, can be attained.

ABOUT THE BOOK

THE INFOGRAPHICS

The colorful information boxes and charts are based on scientific findings that show how applying these habits can have a positive impact on our well-being.

THE GRAY, *Italicized* WRITING

...is taken from the book *The Ministry of Healing,* with occasional adaptation. This book covers topics of practical living such as a healthy home life, healthy relationships with others and with God, and our mental and physical well-being.

HABITS

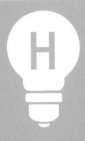

Habits determine our character and destiny. You will see the above lightbulb icons with different habits that can greatly improve your health when put into practice.

DOCTOR SAYS

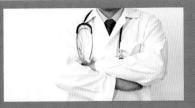

Each chapter has a section called "Doctor Says" in which a medical doctor from Loma Linda gives his thoughts from a medical perspective about the concepts presented.

HENRY & ANNA

You will hear their names mentioned periodically throughout the book. Although this couple is fictitious, their stories are based on various case studies of normal people like us. They may remind you of your neighbor, a friend, an acquaintance, a coworker, a family member, or even yourself.

WHY *THE MINISTRY OF HEALING?*

There is a group of people in Loma Linda, California, who was featured on *U.S. News*, ABC News, twice in *The National Geographic Magazine*, the Oprah Winfrey Show, The Dr. Oz Show, and many other media outlets as one of the people groups that live the longest and the healthiest in the world. This group is composed of many different ethnic groups, so we cannot attribute their good health to good genetics. Their secret? Their lifestyle habits. They identify themselves as Seventh-day Adventist Christians, and these long-living citizens have diligently followed the lifestyle habits outlined in the book, *The Ministry of Healing*.

May you and your loved ones be blessed as you read this book. As you apply the principles presented in these pages, may your physical, mental, emotional, and spiritual health improve greatly. May you experience for yourself that these indeed are habits that heal.

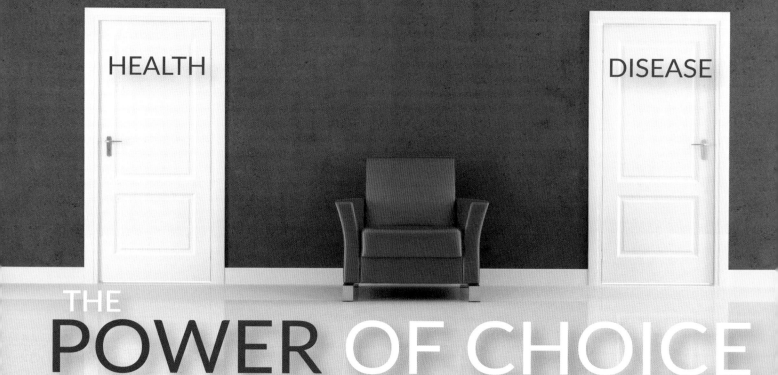

Habit #1

HEALTH

DISEASE

THE POWER OF CHOICE

Henry and Anna didn't make the choice to be healthy earlier in their life. The road to good health begins with making the decision that you want to be healthy. The earlier you make that decision in life, the easier it is to gain good health.

Henry was a football player in high school and ate whatever he wanted, whenever he wanted. Although he stopped playing football soon after graduation, he continued with the same eating habits well into his 40s. It wasn't until his father died from a heart attack that Henry started to consider the impact of his choices. It was not too late for Henry to turn his health around, but it would have been much easier if he had made the decision to be healthy sooner in life.

Choose today that you want to live a healthy life. It is never too early and never too late to decide that you want to be healthy.

The power of the will is not valued as it should be. Let the will be kept awake and rightly directed, and it will impart energy to the whole being and will be a won-
derful aid in the maintenance of health. It is a power also in dealing with disease. Exercised in the right direction, it would control the imagination and be a potent means of resisting and overcoming disease of both mind and body. By the exercise of the will power in placing themselves in right relation to life, patients can do much to cooperate with the physician's efforts for their recovery. There are thousands who can recover health if they will. The Lord does not want them to be sick. He desires them to be well and happy, and they should make up their minds to be well. Often people who seem always to be sick can resist disease simply by refusing to yield to ailments and settle down in a state of inactivity. Rising above their aches and pains, let them engage in useful employment suited to their strength. By such employment and the free use of air and sunlight, many an emaciated sick person might recover health and strength.

The will goes with the labor of the hands; and what these sick people need is to have the will aroused. When the will is dormant, the imagination becomes abnormal, and it is impossible to resist disease. ~ The Ministry of Healing, page 246, 239.

There is great power in the will. But, no matter how determined or how strong-willed a person may be, there are some situations that are very difficult to change. For example, it would not be very logical or compassionate to tell a woman born blind that the reason she cannot see is because she has not determined in her heart to see. This situation may not have much to do with the will or choice. Does this mean that this blind person cannot live a healthy life? No, not at all! There are circumstances we may not be able to change, but there are choices we can make to improve our health. There is a simple, well-known thought, commonly called the Serenity Prayer, that would be beneficial to keep in mind to understand this concept of the power of choice.

"God, grant me the serenity to accept the things I cannot change,
The courage to change the things I can,
And the wisdom to know the difference."

We also need other people to help us get healthier. In the same way as with depression, we must recognize the benefits and our need of being healthy and consciously decide to seek after health.

Life is made up of little decisions. These little decisions are influenced by what we read, what we watch, what we listen to, whom we associate with, and various other factors. Surround yourself with positive people and input good things into your mind.

The use of natural remedies requires an amount of care and effort that many are not willing to give. Nature's process of healing and upbuilding is gradual, and to the impatient it seems slow. The surrender of hurtful indulgences requires sacrifice. But in the end it will be found that nature, unshackled, does her work wisely and well. Those who persevere in obedience to her laws will reap the reward in health of body and health of mind. ~ The Ministry of Healing, page 127.

Not everything in our lives needs to change. There are some things in life that are not within our control to change. However, we can decide to change what needs to be changed. Choose to change what you can to live a healthy life.

God has given us the power of choice; it is ours to exercise. . . . Through the right exercise of the will, an entire change may be made in the life. By yielding up the will to Christ, we ally ourselves with divine power. We receive strength from above to hold us steadfast. A pure and noble life, a life of victory over appetite and lust, is possible to everyone who will unite his weak, wavering human will to the omnipotent, unwavering will of God. ~ The Ministry of Healing, page 176.

Take for example, depression. The first step in treating depression is recognizing that you are depressed. The second step is seeking help[1]. Just as depressed people must recognize their state and choose to seek help, we must recognize our state and decide that we want to be healthy. Just as a depressed person needs others' help to get better, the journey of healthy living cannot be walked alone.

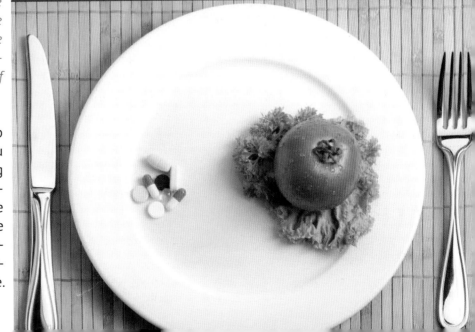

The power of the will is not valued as it should be. Let the will be kept awake and rightly directed, and it will impart energy to the whole being and will be a wonderful aid in the maintenance of health.

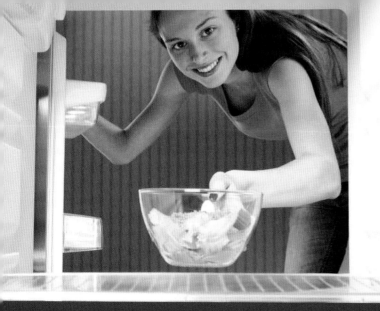

The first step to good health is deciding that you want to be healthy.

Henry and Anna can't remember how many times they've "decided" that they were going to live a healthier life and just one week later they are back to square one. Usually, the first couple days they don't do so badly at sticking to their new regime. However, whether it's cutting back on the potato chips and soda, exercising more, or less time with the TV and Internet, it always seems to become more difficult after a few days.

What we need to realize and remember is that change takes time, patience, and endurance.

During my grade school years, I remember experiencing painfully embarrassing moments in our Wednesday P.E. classes. You see, that's when we had our timed mile runs. Not only was I usually one of the last ones to finish running the mile, but I would periodically pass out from lack of endurance. Needless to say, I did not enjoy running and did not look forward to Wednesdays. Although this memory brings a warm smile to my face now, during this stage of my life where I was overly self-conscious about how I fit in with the rest of the kids, these

moments were literally and figuratively painfully embarrassing.

I remember recounting these moments at school to my father, and being the good father that he is, he firmly stated that he would coach me on running so I could be a strong young lady. I fondly remember some of his tips, such as moving my arms a certain way, breathing in and out, and using the restroom before I ran. But, there is one thing that he told me during one of our running sessions that forever imprinted itself on my heart, mind, and soul. He said, "Many things worth doing in life take time and effort."

What are things worth doing in your life? Whether it's training to have a body strong enough to run or striving everyday toward a healthier life, it will take time and effort. Fast forward about a decade from the days of the running sessions, and I completed my first half-marathon. I ran every inch of the 13.1 miles. The following year, I ran my first full marathon of 26.2 miles. Did it come overnight? No way! I kept up with the tips that my father gave me, and eventually I got better, faster, and even started to enjoy running!

H Make a conscious decision each day to live a healthy life.

So it is with making choices toward a healthier life. You will not achieve a perfectly healthy life overnight. It is the sum of the many choices that you make each and every day that will determine your future. That little school girl who couldn't run one single mile would have been overwhelmed by the thought of one day running 26.2 miles. Likewise, we must not overwhelm ourselves with the ideals we have for our futures. Just as this little school girl took one day at a time, one step at a time, to come to a place where running became enjoyable, we must take one day at a time, one choice at a time, to come to a place where we enjoy living healthfully.

The future of your health depends largely on the choices you make each day. Just as my father gave me tips to be able to run better, this book is designed to give you tips and simple habits that can help you to run this race of life better. The choices you make today will affect your health tomorrow. What will you choose today? The choice is yours.

DOCTOR SAYS
CHOOSE

The first step to good health is deciding that you want to be healthy. Whether you are battling with heart disease, diabetes, cancer, high blood pressure, arthritis, high cholesterol, depression, etc., the first step toward a healthier and happier life is to decide that you want to be healthy and happy.

What we choose on a regular basis turns into habits. Habits form our character, and character determines our destiny. The choices we make on a daily basis are what determine our destiny. So it is with our health. The choices we make will affect our health and determine the outcome of our well-being.

Changing your life to a healthier one can be much like recovering from addictions. It can be difficult and character-building. New habits must replace old habits. You may need to change your surroundings, and even your thoughts and the direction of your will may need to be molded. But the good news is that these choices become easier as they are solidified as habits. As you consistently make good choices, the choices that once seemed so difficult to make become an automatic response. In the end, after all the diligent work, you will be a healthier you! The road to good health is a combination of good choices. Stick to the positive decisions that you make. Do not trade what you want most for what you think you want now. See the next page to help you to make important decisions to live a healthy life.

APPLY IT!

1. Figure out why you want to be healthy. Is it so you can enjoy life to the fullest? Is it so you can see your grandchildren? Is it so you can see your grandchildren graduate from college? Set goals for yourself. List off your reasons for wanting to be healthy:

_____

_____

_____

_____

2. Decide that you want to be healthy. Write a statement of your decision to become healthier.

_____

_____

_____

3. Find other people who want to be healthy like you, and associate with them.
   1. The journey of good health is difficult to be made alone. You need help from others!
   2. Think of the people around you who have similar health goals. Help each other out by keeping each other accountable. Who are those people? List them here:

_____

_____

_____

_____

_____

_____

4. Evaluate your life. Are you heading down the road of good health? Are there certain changes you must make in order to be healthy?
   1. Sometimes it is difficult to figure out what changes would improve your health, and that is why this book was written. Read on to find out more about healthy habits.
   2. What are the changes or improvements that you already know you want/need to make?

_____

_____

_____

5. Write a brief statement below expressing your decision to make the necessary changes to improve your health.

_____

_____

_____

_____

WATER, THE ELIXIR OF LIFE

Why is water necessary?

Water makes up about 60 percent to 70 percent of your body weight.[1, 2] Every system in your body depends on water. For example, water is needed to flush toxins out of vital organs, carry nutrients to your cells, and provide a moist environment for ear, nose, and throat tissues.[3] We cannot go without water for very long. It is estimated that a person can survive without food for a few weeks, but you can only live without water for just a few days.[4, 5]

"Lack of water can lead to dehydration, a condition that occurs when you don't have enough water in your body to carry out normal functions. Even mild dehydration can drain your energy and make you tired." [6]

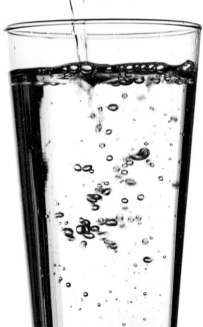

There are many functions of water for your body. Some of those are: regulating body temperature, cushioning and lubricating joints, flushing out waste products, carrying nutrients and oxygen to the cells, and helping dissolve minerals and other nutrients. Water is also important for regulating bowel movements and for keeping the tissues of the mouth, eyes, nose, and skin moistened and hydrated. It also provides protection for the vital organs and the tissues, including the brain and the spinal cord. [7]

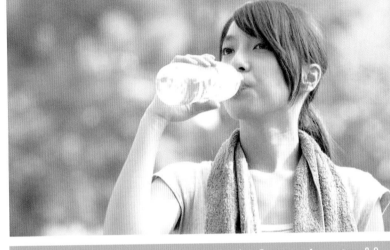

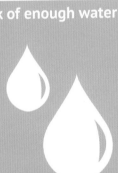

Possible complications from a lack of enough water:[8, 9]
1. Dehydration
2. Intravascular blood clotting
3. Constipation
4. Dizziness
5. Headaches
6. Kidney Stones
7. Gallstones
8. Dry Skin
9. Feeling hungry when your body does not need food
10. Death

In health and in sickness, pure water is one of heaven's choicest blessings. Its proper use promotes health. It is the beverage which God provided to quench the thirst of animals and people. Drunk freely, it helps to supply the necessities of the system and assists nature to resist disease. The external application of water is one of the easiest and most satisfactory ways of regulating the circulation of the blood. A cold or cool bath is an excellent tonic. Warm baths open the pores and thus aid in the elimination of impurities. Both warm and neutral baths soothe the nerves and equalize the circulation. ~ The Ministry of Healing, page 237.

> **"In health and in sickness,** pure water is one of heaven's choicest blessings. **Its proper use promotes health."**

Water is an absolute necessity for good health. Now, can any type of liquid do?

Caffeine
Caffeinated drinks often do more harm than good in the long run. (See Habit #10.) Caffeinated drinks can be worse for you since they act as diuretics, meaning they can dehydrate you more than hydrate you.

Sweet Drinks
Consumption of sweetened beverages has been shown to cause an increased risk of obesity, type 2 diabetes, metabolic syndrome, heart disease, gout, and kidney stones. Recent studies are now showing that sweetened beverages instead of water may even increase the risk of getting hypertension. [10]

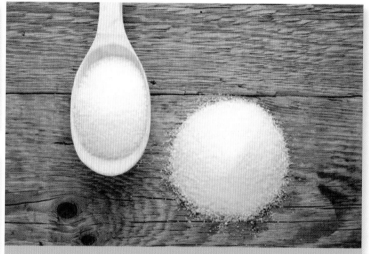

Sodas:
a. High in sugar and calories
b. Has potentially harmful chemicals for coloring and/or artificial sweetening
c. Caffeinated

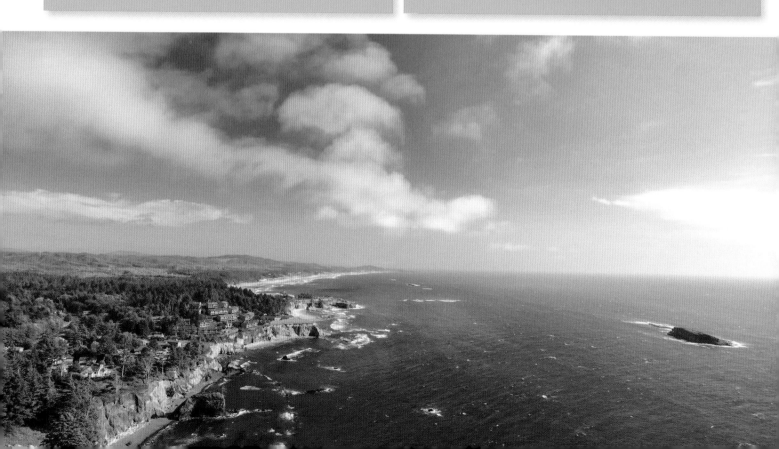

But many have never learned by experience the beneficial effects of the proper use of water, and they are afraid of it. Water treatments are not appreciated as they should be, and to apply them skillfully requires work that many are unwilling to perform. There are many ways in which water can be applied to relieve pain and check disease. All should become intelligent in its use in simple home treatments. Parents, especially, should know how to care for their families in both health and sickness. ~ The Ministry of Healing, page 237.

For your safety and well-being, please consult a medical professional when injuries, burns, or other maladies occur, but here are some common ways to use water to alleviate ailments.

1 Hot-and-cold contrast showers [11]

Many people like to alternate the water temperature from hot to cold to increase their circulation. (This may not be advisable for a person-feeling faint.) You will not only feel good with proper blood circulation, but good circulation can prevent 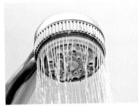 many illnesses and help maintain good health. A commonly suggested formula is three minutes hot water then thirty seconds cold water. Repeat three times and end on cold. This suggested formula can easily be adjusted to your comfort level.

2 Hot-and-cold towels [12]

As mentioned above, proper blood circulation can help with many things, including simple muscle aches. Some people like to alternate applying towels dipped in hot water and cold water to their sore muscles to improve blood flow. Be careful not to 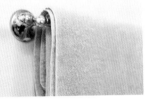 burn yourself! Caution is necessary, especially for people with diabetes or those whose nerves have been damaged by injury or surgery.

3 Ice or Cold Compresses

Applying ice or something cold can help alleviate pain or swelling in some minor injuries such as sprained ankles and stubbed 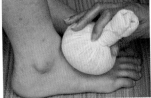 fingers. It can also help with minor burns. Again, use discretion and consult a medical professional if needed.

4 Baths

Herbal baths, bubble baths, and aromatic baths—these can all be very relaxing. Soaking in a tub full of nicely scented warm water or just simply warm water can be very calming and stress-relieving.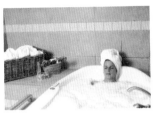

5 Foot baths

Soaking your feet in clean, warm water can also have a calming effect on some as well. It can be especially beneficial for diabetics to clean their feet routinely as they can have a decreased sensation and can be more prone to developing cuts, bruises, and infections.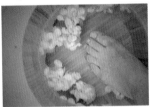

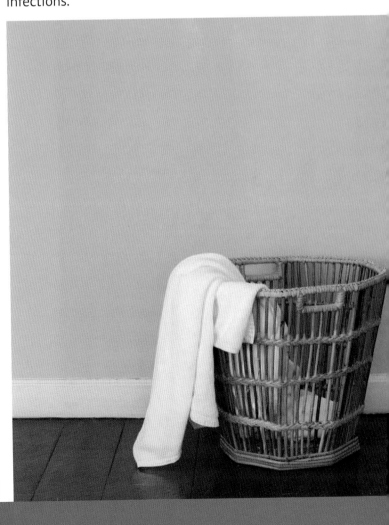

Feeling like you're going under the weather?
1. Drink plenty of water.

2. Take a refreshing shower or a soothing bath.

Most persons would receive benefit from a cool or tepid bath every day, morning or evening. Instead of increasing the liability to take cold, a bath, properly taken, fortifies against cold, because it improves the circulation; the blood is brought to the surface, and a more easy and regular flow is obtained. The mind and the body are alike invigorated. The muscles become more flexible, the intellect is made brighter. The bath is a soother of the nerves. Bathing helps the bowels, the stomach, and the liver, giving health and energy to each, and it promotes digestion. ~ The Ministry of Healing, page 276.

Water is not only good for you to drink and consume, but also to bathe with as well! Daily showers or baths will not only keep you clean but will also help to improve blood circulation, as mentioned above.

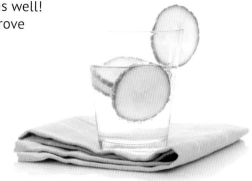

DOCTOR SAYS

The ideal amount of water to drink will vary from person to person and with individual circumstances. Some may need more than this depending on their circumstances, such as activity level and the climate of the area. This is a general formula that will differ from person to person.

How much water to drink?*	
100 lbs	50 oz (6-7 glasses of water)**
130 lbs	65 oz (8-9 glasses of water)**
150 lbs	75 oz (9-10 glasses of water)**
180 lbs	90 oz (11-12 glasses of water)**
200 lbs+	100 oz+ (12+ glasses of water)**

*Half of your weight in ounces. Your weight (in lbs)/2 = amount of water to drink daily.
**Calculated based on 8-oz glasses.

1. It is better to drink between meals. Avoid drinking excessive amounts of water with your meals.
2. Another practical way to figure out if you're drinking enough water is by the color and smell of your urine. The lighter the color and less odor there is, the more hydrated you are. The darker and stronger the smell, the more dehydrated you are. **Disclaimer:** *Some medications and/or supplements may change the color and smell of your urine regardless of the amount of water you drink.*
3. If you have a hard time drinking plain water, try adding a wedge of lemon or other fruits or vegetables. (Cucumbers or strawberries are two of my favorites.)

Habit #3

NO EXERCISE,
KNOW SICKNESS

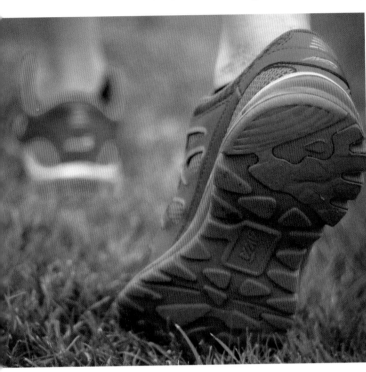

Action is a law of our being. Every organ of the body has its appointed work, upon the performance of which its development and strength depend. The normal action of all the organs gives strength and vigor, while the tendency of disuse is toward decay and death. Bind up an arm, even for a few weeks, then free it from its bands, and you will see that it is weaker than the one you have been using moderately during the same time. Inactivity produces the same effect upon the whole muscular system.

Inactivity is a fruitful cause of disease. Exercise quickens and equalizes the circulation of the blood, but in idleness the blood does not circulate freely, and the changes in it, so necessary to life and health, do not take place. The skin, too, becomes inactive. Impurities are not expelled as they would be if the circulation had been quickened by vigorous exercise, the skin kept in a healthy condition, and the lungs fed with plenty of pure, fresh air. This state of the system throws a double burden on the excretory organs, and disease is the result.

Ministers, teachers, students, and other brain workers often suffer from illness as the result of severe mental taxation, unrelieved by physical exercise. What these persons need is a more active life. Strictly temperate habits, combined with proper exercise, would ensure both mental and physical vigor, and would give power of endurance to all brain workers.

Those who have overtaxed their physical powers should not be encouraged to forgo manual labor entirely. But labor, to be of the greatest advantage, should be systematic and agreeable. Outdoor exercise is the best; it should be so planned as to strengthen by use the organs that have become weakened; and the heart should be in it; the labor of the hands should never degenerate into mere drudgery.

When the long-term sick have nothing to occupy their time and attention, their thoughts become centered upon themselves, and they grow morbid and irritable. Many times they dwell upon their bad feelings until they think themselves much worse than they really are and wholly unable to do anything.

In all these cases well-directed physical exercise would prove an effective remedial agent. In some cases it is indispensable to the recovery of health. The will goes with the labor of the hands; and what they need is to have the will aroused. When the will is dormant, the imagination becomes abnormal, and it is impossible to resist disease.

Inactivity is the greatest curse that could come upon most of the chronically ill. Light employment in useful labor, while it does not tax mind or body, has a happy influence upon both. It strengthens the muscles, improves the circulation, and gives the person the satisfaction of knowing that he is not wholly useless in this busy world. He may be able to do but little at first, but he will soon find his strength increasing, and the amount of work done can be increased accordingly.

"Action is a law of our being....Inactivity is a fruitful cause of disease."

Exercise aids the person with indigestion by giving the digestive organs a healthy tone. To engage in severe study or violent physical exercise immediately after eating, hinders the work of digestion; but a short walk after a meal, with the head erect and the shoulders back, is a great benefit.

Notwithstanding all that is said and written concerning its importance, there are still many who neglect physical exercise. Some grow obese because the system is clogged; others become thin and feeble because their vital powers are exhausted in disposing of an excess of food. The liver is burdened in its effort to cleanse the blood of impurities, and illness is the result.

Those whose habits are sedentary should, when the weather will permit, exercise in the open air every day, summer or winter.

Such exercise would in many cases be better for the health than medicine. Physicians often advise their patients to take an ocean voyage, to go to some mineral spring, or to visit different places for change of climate, when in most cases if they would eat temperately, and take cheerful, healthful exercise, they would recover health and would save time and money. ~ The Ministry of Healing, pages 237-240.

BENEFITS OF EXERCISE [1,2]

THE BENEFITS OF EXERCISING REGULARLY ARE COUNTLESS, BUT HERE ARE A FEW:

- Lower risk of early death
- Lower risk of coronary heart disease
- Lower risk of stroke
- Lower risk of high blood pressure
- Lower risk of type 2 diabetes
- Lower risk of colon, breast, endometrial, and lung cancers
- Improved bone health
- Improved cardiorespiratory and muscular fitness

- Improved sleep quality
- Improved digestion and elimination
- Improved total cholesterol
- Greater joint flexibility
- Reduced symptoms of depression
- Better cognitive function
- Healthier body weight
- Healthier skin
- Less flu and fewer colds

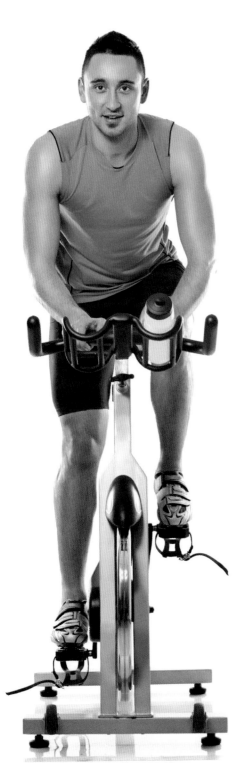

Exercise would in many cases do more than medicine to improve one's health.

SOME OF THE BENEFITS OF EXERCISE EXPLAINED:

1 Stress Management

Exercise can cause a release of chemicals called endorphins. "These chemicals give you a feeling of happiness and positively affect your overall sense of well-being." [3]

2 Bone Strength

"An active lifestyle benefits bone density. Regular weight-bearing exercise promotes bone formation, delays bone loss and may protect against osteoporosis." [4]

3 Stronger Immune System

"Regular moderate exercise may have a beneficial effect on the immune function. The findings from some studies support the possibility that exercise may delay immunosenescence, age dependent decline in immune function" [5]

4 Back Pain Remedy

"By increasing muscle strength and endurance and improving flexibility and posture, regular exercise helps to prevent back pain." [6]

5 Improved Memory and Learning Abilities

"Exercise stimulates the formation of new brain cells (neurons). Also, exercise strengthens connections between those cells. The areas of the brain that are stimulated through exercise are associated with memory and learning." [7]

6 Improved Mental Function for all Age Groups

"Physical activity improves cognitive performance, information processing and may delay cognitive impairment and dementia. For instance, older adults who engage in regular physical activity have better performances in tests implying decision-making process, memory and problem solving. And what about children? University of Illinois researchers have found that physical activity may enhance the academic achievements of children by improving their attention and working memory skills." [8]

Exercise is one of the habits that can make up for a lot of other bad habits or lack of good habits. For example, Henry was able to eat whatever he wanted whenever he wanted when he was younger without gaining a pound, partly because he was a very active athlete. There were other factors such as he was younger and had better metabolism that allowed him to eat limitlessly without seeming to gain any fat, but exercise definitely helped him to burn the calories off.

One article published in the *Time* magazine featured a study in which the findings showed that the lack of exercise caused as many premature deaths as smoking! Here is an excerpt from the article:

"About 5.3 million of the 57 million deaths worldwide in 2008 could be attributed to inactivity, the new report estimates, largely due to four major diseases: heart disease, Type 2 diabetes, breast cancer and colon cancer. The study finds that if physical inactivity could be reduced by just 10%, it could avert some 533,000 deaths a year; if reduced by 25%, 1.3 million deaths could be prevented." [9]

Although exercise can help make up for the other bad habits or lack of good habits, that does not mean that it is okay for us to disregard the health laws. These habits together bring health and healing and help us to achieve optimal health.

Now that you have seen the great positive effects of exercise and the great negative effects that can stem from a lack of it, what next? Many people have a difficult time sticking to their commitment of exercising regularly. So, here are some suggestions to help:

1. Schedule It

Why do we not think twice about keeping a doctor's appointment or other important appointment? One reason is that it is scheduled. We mark it down in our calendars or put it into our phones. We take a mental note of it ahead of time rather than try to go to the doctor's when it's convenient for us to go. We work out our other daily engagements around it. We make time for it. We put it high on our priority list to keep these important appointments. That is how we should treat our exercise times. It is very important for your health. Schedule it into your daily routine.

2. Multi-task While Exercising

A very common answer as to why someone may not exercise on a regular basis is the lack of enough time for it. The American culture today seems to embrace this constant desire to do as much as possible in the least amount of time possible. The average American today seems to have very much to do in very little time. Therefore, think of some things that you could do while exercising to maximize your time and maybe give yourself something to look forward to, such as listening to audiobooks or talking to a friend or loved one on the phone while walking or jogging.

3. Exercise in Groups

Having an accountability partner makes keeping our commitments much easier. Whether it's a running buddy or joining a fitness class with twenty other people, having other people doing the same thing with you can increase your motivation to stick with it. Plus, having other people around could make it seem like a fun social event.

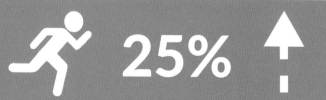

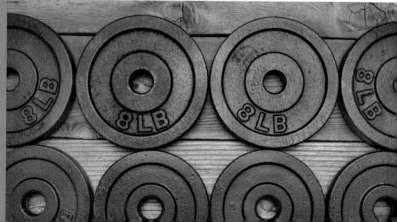

25%

If physical activity was increased by just 25%, 1.3 million deaths could be prevented.

MAKE IT A LIFESTYLE

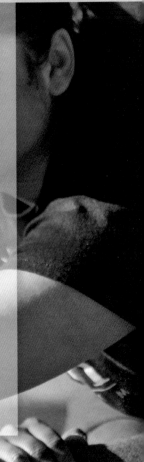

- Sit on an exercise ball instead of a chair. This will give you better posture and cause your abdominal muscles to work more.

- Take the stairs instead of the elevator.

- Don't try to find the closest parking spot, rather find a parking spot farther away so you will have to walk more.

- Try carrying your groceries from the store to your car rather than taking them in a cart.

- When grocery shopping, try using the basket instead of the cart.

- Consider having a meeting while you walk if it's only two or three people. This works great, too, if you simply want to chat with a loved one!

- Take up gardening

- View any sort of waiting time as your golden opportunity to exercise!!

  - Do wall push-ups or stretches while waiting for the copy/fax machine.

  - Stretch out your neck and shoulders while waiting at a red light.

  - Stand up and walk around every time you are on the phone.

4. Do a Type of Exercise You Enjoy

Find an exercise that you don't view as drudgery. Some people enjoy playing team sports. Others enjoy a brisk hike in the woods. Others may enjoy gardening, chopping wood, or feeling productive while exercising. There are a myriad of activities available. If you have not found the exercise that fits your niche, keep trying out different activities. Have fun while exercising!

5. Live an Active Lifestyle

The easiest way not to skip out on your exercising is to incorporate it into your life. Although having a set time in which we exercise vigorously can greatly benefit our health, sometimes we are not always able to do that. See the list above for some ideas to stay active even while at work, at home, or simply running errands.

Henry and Anna could improve their health greatly if they followed the above concepts. They could enroll in an exercise group or class. They could take up gardening or incorporate some of the suggestions for an active lifestyle. They could have "exercise dates" together and take turns doing the kinds of exercising that they each like.

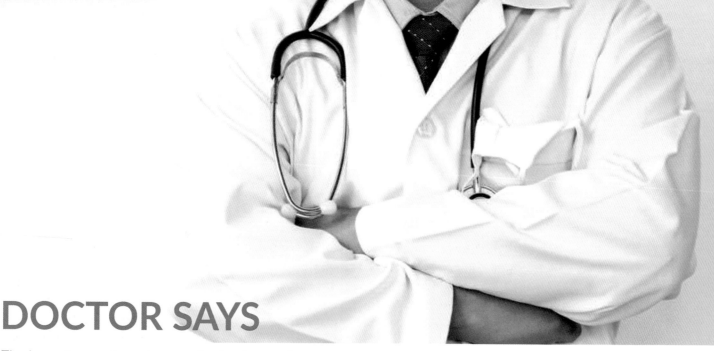

DOCTOR SAYS

The importance of regular exercise is often underestimated. Proper exercise could in many cases do *more* than proper food choices to improve one's health.

- Especially harmful is sitting for long periods of time with no breaks. Consider getting a high table if you need to so you can stand and work.

- Walking is a great form of exercise. Taking fifteen to thirty-minute walks after meals could make a world of difference. Even if you cannot walk, you can still exercise. Start by moving what you can— your arms, legs, or anything that you can move.

- Exercise, exercise, and exercise!! But avoid injury!

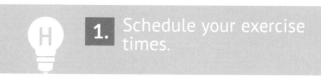

1. Schedule your exercise times.

2. Do types of exercise that you enjoy.

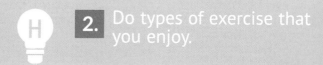

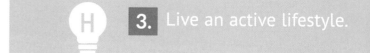

3. Live an active lifestyle.

TESTIMONIAL

Maddy

During her third year of college, Maddy realized that she needed help with depression. She went to a ten-day depression recovery program, implemented the things she was taught to overcome this disease, and is happy to say that she is a brand-new person! But the road was not as short or easy as it sounds.

Maddy was sexually abused as a young child and struggled with insomnia, pain from several sports injuries,

I am no longer depressed. Sure, I may have difficult days and feel upset just like everybody else, but overall on a daily basis I'm content.

and a poor self-image throughout her life. She eventually developed depression but masked it behind her good grades, athleticism, musical talents, and other outwardly positive achievements. Eating also became a way of finding control in her life. She craved sweets because of the good feeling she got while eating them. To find personal worth, she would overwork herself mercilessly to become a high achiever. Others were amazed that she was so good at everything she did, but underneath it all was a hurting heart, struggling to find self-worth and freedom from depression.

At the depression recovery program, Maddy received counseling to correct her self-destructive way of thinking as well as to find her self-worth in Jesus Christ. Doctors ran tests and figured out different ways for her to find balance physically and also in other aspects of her life.

She was put on a very structured schedule, going to bed at 9:00 P.M. and waking up at 6:00 A.M. She went on a strictly plant-based diet and ate lots of foods rich in tryptophan and omega-3s, such as flax seeds, beans, walnuts, kale, and other fresh fruits and vegetables. She stayed away from using laptops, smartphones, and other electronics during the program. She exercised vigorously, spending two to three hours a day walking and hiking in the beautiful outdoors, breathing in the crisp, fresh air. She also underwent water treatments, in which she alternately immersed herself in hot and cold water to improve her blood circulation, especially to her brain.

Through these good lifestyle habits, counseling, and spiritual activities, Maddy started to feel the fogginess in her mind lift, her physical pain decreased, and she started to hope for recovery. The program itself was only ten days long, but she was instructed and equipped to carry out these habits in her everyday life. Although living by these good habits was much more difficult outside of the program, she persevered and diligently followed the recovery plan prescribed by her doctors with one goal in mind—recovering from depression.

With help from loved ones and by the grace of God, Maddy has recovered from depression. She says, "I am no longer depressed. Sure, I may have difficult days and feel upset just like everybody else, but overall on a daily basis I'm content. I no longer have that heavy weight on my chest anymore. The experience that I've had I've been able to share with others and help others who are struggling with depression." Today, Maddy does just that. She finds great joy in serving Jesus and helping others find that same peace and joy that she has found.

REST IS BEST

Pure air, sunlight, abstemiousness, rest, exercise, proper diet, the use of water, trust in divine power—these are the true remedies.
~The Ministry of Healing, page 127.

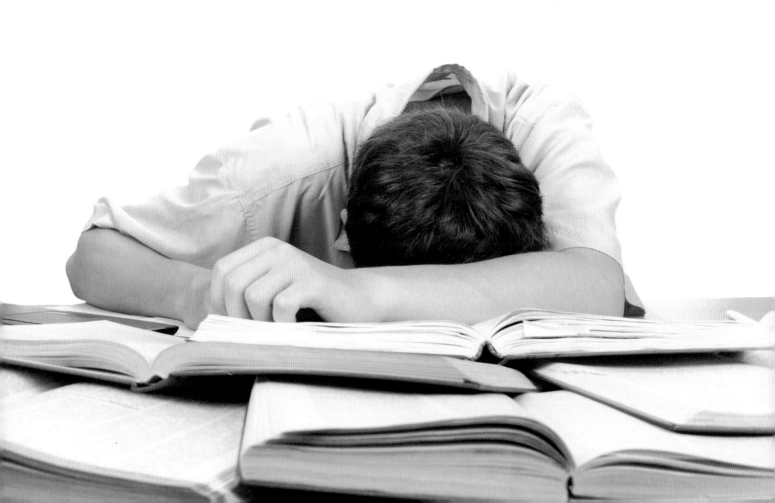

Henry and Anna usually both get about six hours of sleep on an average night. They both drink coffee throughout the day to stay alert and awake. They don't see a problem with this lifestyle. They don't think that it is necessary for them to get more quality sleep at night, since their problem of drowsiness could be solved with drinking some caffeine. But what they don't realize is that the purpose of getting good quality sleep is more than just having energy for the day. The quality and the quantity of sleep could affect your weight, risk of disease, skin, mental, emotional, and spiritual well-being, and many other aspects of your health. Read on to learn more.

In order to understand why we need a proper amount of sleep for good health, it is helpful to know what actually happens when we sleep.

What happens when we sleep?
In short, during sleep our bodies repair, rejuvenate, and grow. Sleep is important for a healthy brain function, a healthy body, and it is a time for children and teens to grow.[1]

There are 5 stages of sleep[2]
Stage 1: The lightest stage of sleep. This is the stage between being awake and falling asleep.

Stage 2: This is the onset of sleep. You start to become disengaged from your surroundings and your body temperature tends to drop.

Stages 3 and 4: These stages are the deepest and the most restorative sleep. Blood pressure drops, breathing becomes slower, muscles relax, blood supply to muscles increases, tissue growth and repair occur, energy is restored, and hormones are released. When people are awakened during these stages they may feel groggy or disoriented for a few minutes. Some children may experience bedwetting, night terrors, or sleepwalking during these stages.

REM sleep: Known as the Rapid Eye Movement stage because the eyes dart back and forth. During this stage the brain is active and dreams occur. The body becomes immobile and relaxed, so people do not act out their dreams. This stage typically occurs about ninety minutes after falling asleep.

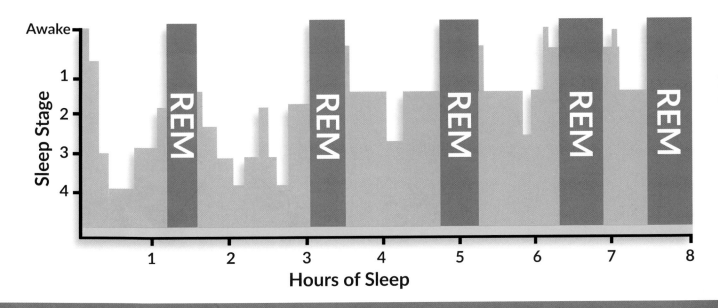

Although sleep patterns will vary from person-to-person, a typical cycle through the stages of sleep may look like the above chart. We enter into REM sleep about seventy to ninety minutes after we fall asleep and tend to cycle through the first two stages and REM sleep as we get closer to the morning. [3]

WHY IS SLEEP IMPORTANT?

Lack of sufficient sleep or low-quality sleep has been connected to many problems and ailments. Here are some of the common risks associated with sleep problems.

1. Obesity [4, 5]

Sleep deprivation has been associated with lower levels of leptin, a hormone that signals the brain that it has had enough food and is full, and higher levels of ghrelin, another hormone that stimulates appetite. As a result, we have a body that does not

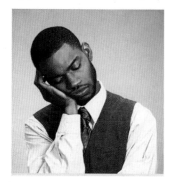

easily notice when it's had enough to eat and has a higher desire to eat more. In addition to this physiological change, when we don't get enough sleep, we simply may be too tired to exercise to go burn off those extra calories.

2. Increased risk of disease

Studies have shown that insufficient sleep can alter the way the body processes glucose, which can lead to diabetes.[6] Another study which simulated the disturbed sleep patterns of shift workers on healthy, young adults showed that in as little as four days, 30 percent of them had sugar levels that qualified them as pre-diabetic.[7]

POOR SLEEP IS LINKED TO
A HIGHER RISK OF...[8, 9]

- Diabetes
- Heart disease
- Kidney disease
- Hypertension
- Strokes

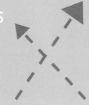

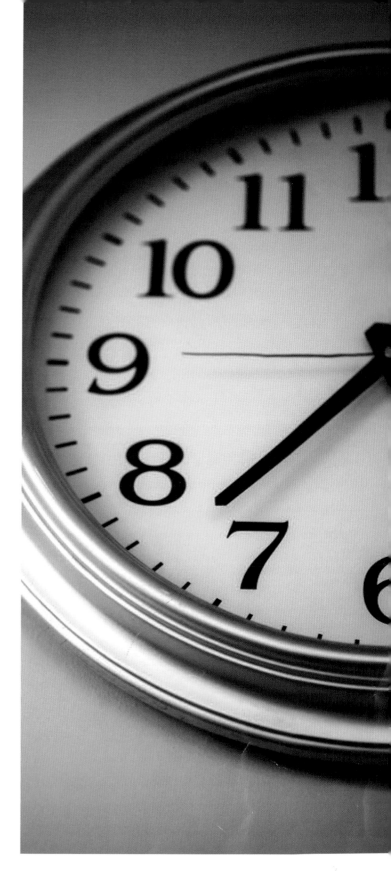

3. Lowered immune system response

Numerous research studies have indicated that the more sleep deprived we become, the less the immune system is able to do its job. Our bodies become less able to fight off colds, flu, and even infections.[10, 11]

4. Mood disorders

We all have experienced it—some more than others. We go to bed late or pull an all-nighter trying to meet that deadline or studying for that test and the next day, we feel drained—physically and emotionally. Many people become more irritable, have more mood swings, have difficulty getting along with others, and feel more stressed. Other behaviors may include anger, sadness, difficulty paying attention, and/or feeling impulsive. Long-term sleep deficiency has been linked to other severe disorders such as: depression, suicide, and other risk-taking behavior. [12]

5. Higher risk of injury

Sleep deprivation has been linked to many notorious disasters, like the destruction of the space shuttle Challenger, the grounding of the Exxon Valdez, nuclear explosions, and other occupational errors. Studies also indicate that more than one out of five auto accidents in the United States results from drowsy driving. That's about one million crashes a year that could be prevented if we just got the sleep we needed.[13] When we are overly tired, we are more likely to trip, fall down the stairs, or cut ourselves while preparing dinner. Accidents like these could have serious consequences.

6. Impaired mental function

We have all felt it at one point or another. Our minds just feel slower when we do not get enough sleep. Studies have shown that when we get good sleep, our learning ability and our problem-solving skills are enhanced. It also helps us to pay attention better, make decisions more easily, and be more creative.[14] When we don't get enough sleep, we are more likely to make odd mistakes, like leaving our keys in the refrigerator by accident. [15]

Even our memory is affected by our sleep. "Studies have shown that while we sleep, our brains process and consolidate our memories from the day."[16] When we don't get enough sleep, it seems as if those memories may not get stored correctly, or may be lost entirely.

SABBATH REST

One other thing that the long-living Seventh-day Adventists practice is following the Bible Sabbath. From Friday sunset to Saturday sunset, they take this 24-hour period to rest. This does not mean they are sleeping all day long, but they take time to refresh and rejuvenate from the week's work. Many Seventh-day Adventists enjoy time with friends and family, attend church, and worship God during this time. They take time to seek physical, mental, emotional, and spiritual rest. See Habit #7 for more information about the Sabbath.

Jesus looked upon the distressed and heart-burdened, those whose hopes were blighted, and who with

SUGGESTIONS FOR GETTING GOOD SLEEP: [17,18]

1. **Exercise during the daytime.**
Daily exercise often helps people sleep, although rigorous exercising right before bedtime can interfere with falling asleep.

2. **Keep your bedroom dark and at an even temperature.**

3. **Put away/turn off laptops, computer screens, tablets, cell phones, and any other electronic devices when preparing for bedtime.**

4. **Stick to a regular bedtime and wake time every day, even on weekends.**

5. **Avoid caffeine, alcohol, and nicotine.**

6. **Avoid late-night meals and snacks.**
Your body will have to continue to digest into the night, making it more difficult for you to get good, quality sleep.

7. **Don't lie in bed awake.**
If you can't fall asleep, don't just lie in bed. Get up and do something else until you feel tired. The stress of not being able to fall asleep can actually contribute to insomnia.

8. **Have a relaxing routine before going to bed.**
Whether it's taking a warm bath, reading, meditating, journaling, or praying, having a routine of restful activities can condition your body to sleep better.

earthly joys were seeking to quiet the longing of the soul, and He invited all to find rest in Him.

Tenderly He invited the toiling people, "Take My yoke upon you, and learn of Me; for I am meek and lowly in heart: and ye shall find rest unto your souls." Matthew 11:29.

In these words, Christ was speaking to every human being. Whether they know it or not, all are weary and heavy-laden. All are weighed down with burdens that only Christ can remove. The heaviest burden that we bear is the burden of sin. If we were left to bear this burden, it would crush us. But the Sinless One has taken our place. "The Lord hath laid on Him the iniquity of us all." Isaiah 53:6.

He has borne the burden of our guilt. He will take the load from our weary shoulders. He will give us rest. The burden of care and sorrow also He will bear. He invites us to cast all our care upon Him; for He carries us upon His heart.

> "Take My yoke upon you, and learn of Me; for I am meek and lowly in heart: and ye shall find rest unto your souls."
> ~ Matthew 11:29

The Elder Brother of our race is by the eternal throne. He looks upon every soul who is turning his face toward Him as the Savior. He knows by experience what are the weaknesses of humanity, what are our wants, and where lies the strength of our temptations; for He was "in all points tempted like as we are, yet without sin." Hebrews 4:15. He is watching over you, trembling child of God. Are you tempted? He will deliver. Are you weak? He will strengthen. Are you ignorant? He will enlighten. Are you wounded? He will heal. The Lord "telleth the number of the stars;" and yet "He healeth the broken in heart, and bindeth up their wounds." Psalm 147:4, 3.

Whatever your anxieties and trials, spread out your case before the Lord. Your spirit will be braced for endurance. The way will be open for you to disentangle yourself from embarrassment and difficulty. The weaker and more helpless you know yourself to be, the stronger will you become in His strength. The heavier your burdens, the more blessed the rest in casting them upon your Burden Bearer.

Circumstances may separate friends; the restless waters of the wide sea may roll between us and them. But no circumstances, no distance, can separate us from the Savior. Wherever we may be, He is at our right hand, to support, maintain, uphold, and cheer. Greater than the love of a mother for her child is Christ's love for His redeemed. It is our privilege to rest in His love, to say, "I will trust Him; for He gave His life for me."

Human love may change, but Christ's love knows no change. When we cry to Him for help, His hand is stretched out to save. ~The Ministry of Healing, pages 71, 72.

> "For the mountains shall depart, and the hills be removed; but my kindness shall not depart from thee, neither shall the covenant of my peace be removed, saith the LORD that hath mercy on thee." ~ Isaiah 54:10

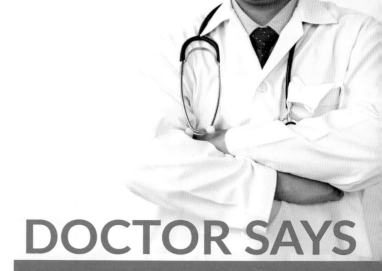

DOCTOR SAYS

Getting daily, weekly, monthly, and annual rest is very important.

- **Daily:** Sleeping at proper times at night and taking naps if necessary.
- **Weekly:** Taking one day out of the week, the Sabbath, to rest.
- **Monthly/Annual:** Vacations

For optimum health, avoid working night shifts and swing shifts as much as possible.

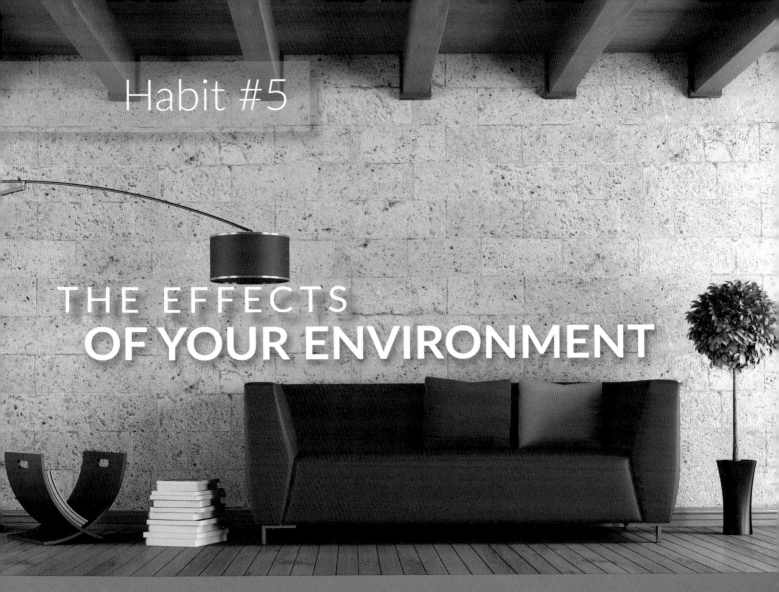

Habit #5

THE EFFECTS
OF YOUR ENVIRONMENT

Instead of dwelling where only human works can be seen, where the sights and sounds frequently suggest thoughts of evil, where turmoil and confusion bring weariness and tension, go where you can look upon the works of God. Find rest of spirit in the beauty and quietude and peace of nature. Let the eye rest on the green fields, the groves, and the hills. Look up to the blue sky, unobscured by the city's dust and smoke, and breathe the invigorating air of heaven. ~ The Ministry of Healing, *page 367.*

Henry and Anna, like many Americans, spend most of their day indoors. They drive through traffic-jammed, smog-filled highways to get to a desk or cubicle inside an office building. There's not much nature to speak of in their neighborhood other than the front lawn and some dirt in their backyard. Their weekends usually consist of sleeping in, watching TV, eating out, some shopping, and an occasional movie.

Life wasn't always like this, though. In their younger years, Henry was an athletic, outdoors-type of guy. He had a core group of friends that he would go mountain climbing, camping, or simply play basketball with. Anna wasn't as athletic, but she too enjoyed being outdoors with their small children. She fondly remembers times at the park with other young mothers as their children played happily on the swings and in the sandbox. But life has taken a toll on them. With credit card bills and the expenses of raising children, Anna has gone back to work, and their leisurely time in the great outdoors has diminished. Their nice home always used to be so clean, fresh, and inviting, but now even the household chores have been somewhat neglected. Although it may seem difficult for them at first, if they would adjust their lives to incorporate more time in nature and choose their surroundings well, they would experience positive health benefits.

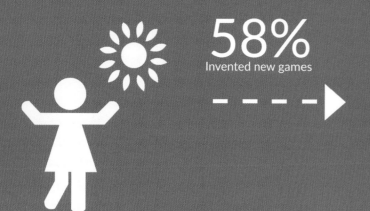

58%
Invented new games

- - - - ➤

According to a study conducted by Danish researchers, 58% of the kindergarteners connected with the outdoors showed more creativity by inventing new games versus only 16% of the indoor kindergarteners who invented new games.[1]

The Creator chose for our first parents the surroundings best adapted for their health and happiness. He did not place them in a palace or surround them with the artificial adornments and luxuries that so many today are struggling to obtain. He placed them in close touch with nature and in close communion with the holy ones of heaven.

In the garden that God prepared as a home for His children, graceful shrubs and delicate flowers greeted the eye at every turn. There were trees of every variety, many of them heavy with fragrant and delicious fruit. On their branches the birds caroled their songs of praise. Under their shadow the creatures of the earth sported together without a fear.

Adam and Eve, in their untainted purity, delighted in the sights and sounds of Eden. God appointed them their work in the garden, "to dress it and to keep it." Genesis 2:15. Each day's labor brought them health and gladness, and the happy pair greeted with joy the visits of their Creator, as in the cool of the day He walked and talked with them. Daily God taught them His lessons.

The plan of life which God appointed for our first parents has lessons for us. Although sin has cast its shadow over the earth, God desires His children to find delight in the works of His hands. The more closely His plan of life is followed, the more wonderfully will He work to restore suffering humanity. The sick need to be brought into close touch with nature. An outdoor life amid natural surroundings would work wonders for many a helpless and almost hopeless sick person.

The noise and excitement and confusion of the cities, their cramped and artificial life, are most wearisome and exhausting to the sick. The air, heavy with smoke and dust, with poisonous gases, and with germs of disease, is a peril to life. The sick, for the most part shut within four walls, come almost to feel as if they were prisoners in their rooms. They look out on houses and pavements and hurrying crowds, with perhaps not even a glimpse of blue sky or sunshine, of grass or flower or tree. Shut up in this way, they brood over their suffering and sorrow, and become a prey to their own sad thoughts.

And for those who are weak in moral power, the cities abound in dangers. In them, patients who have unnatural appetites to overcome are continually exposed to temptation. They need to be placed amid new surroundings where the current of their thoughts will be changed; they need to be placed under influences entirely different from those that have wrecked their lives. Let them for a while be removed from those influences that lead away from God, into a purer atmosphere.

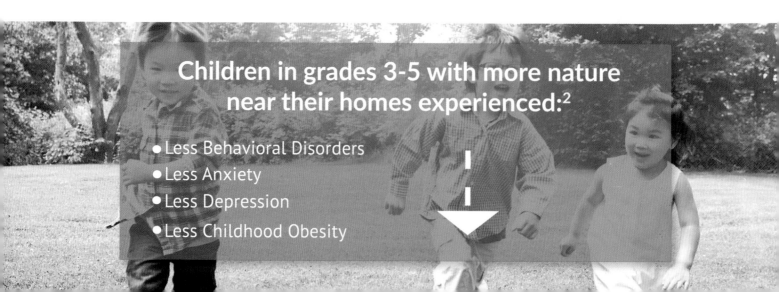

Children in grades 3-5 with more nature near their homes experienced:[2]

- Less Behavioral Disorders
- Less Anxiety
- Less Depression
- Less Childhood Obesity

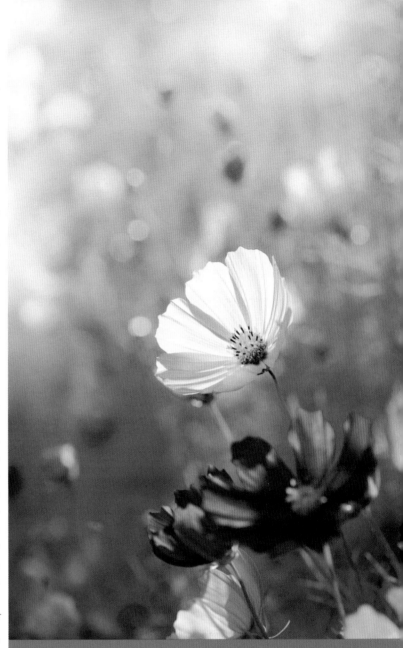

Institutions for the care of the sick would be far more successful if they could be established away from the cities. And so far as possible, all who are seeking to recover health should place themselves amid country surroundings where they can have the benefit of outdoor life. Nature is God's physician. The pure air, the glad sunshine, the flowers and trees, the orchards and vineyards, and outdoor exercise amid these surroundings, are health-giving, life-giving.

Physicians and nurses should encourage their patients to be much in the open air. Outdoor life is the only remedy that many of the chronically sick need. It has a wonderful power to heal diseases caused by the excitements and excesses of fashionable life, a life that weakens and destroys the powers of body, mind, and soul.

How glad would such sick people be to sit in the open air, rejoice in the sunshine, and breathe the fragrance of tree and flower! There are life-giving properties in the balsam of the pine, in the fragrance of the cedar and the fir, and other trees also have properties that are health restoring.

To the chronically sick, nothing so tends to restore health and happiness as living amid attractive country surroundings. Here the most helpless ones can sit or lie in the sunshine or in the shade of the trees. They have only to lift their eyes to see above them the beautiful foliage. A sweet sense of restfulness and refreshing comes over them as they listen to the murmuring of the breezes. The drooping spirits revive. The waning strength is regained. Unconsciously the mind becomes peaceful, the fevered pulse more calm and regular. As the sick grow stronger, they will venture to take a few steps to gather some of the lovely flowers, precious messengers of God's love to His afflicted family here below.

Plans should be devised for keeping patients out of doors. For those who are able to work, let some pleasant, easy employment be provided. Show them how agreeable and helpful this outdoor work is. Encourage them to breathe the fresh air. Teach them to breathe deeply, and in breathing and speaking to exercise the abdominal muscles. This is an education that will be invaluable to them.

Exercise in the open air should be prescribed as a life-giving necessity. And for such exercises there is nothing better than the cultivation of the soil. Let patients have flower beds to care for, or work to do in the orchard or vegetable garden. As they are encouraged to leave their rooms and spend time in the open air, cultivating flowers or doing some other light, pleasant work, their attention will be diverted from themselves and their sufferings.

The more the patients can be kept out of doors, the less care will they require. The more cheerful their surroundings, the more helpful will they be. Shut up in the house, be it ever so elegantly furnished, they will grow fretful and gloomy. Surround them with the beautiful things of nature; place them where they can see the flowers growing and hear

Some Restorative Benefits of Nature[3]

- Lower Blood Pressure
- Boosted Immune Function
- Reduced Stress
- Quicker Recovery from Surgeries
- Lower Anxiety
- Less Need for Pain Medication in Hospital Patients
- Overall Improved Mood [4]

Nature is God's physician. The pure air, the glad sunshine, the flowers and trees, the orchards and vineyards, and outdoor exercise amid these surroundings, are health-giving, life-giving.

the birds singing, and their hearts will break into song in harmony with the songs of the birds. Relief will come to body and mind. The intellect will be awakened, the imagination quickened, and the mind prepared to appreciate the beauty of God's word.

In nature may always be found something to divert the attention of the sick from themselves and direct their thoughts to God. Surrounded by His wonderful works, their minds are uplifted from the things that are seen to the things that are unseen. The beauty of nature leads them to think of the heavenly home, where there will be nothing to mar the loveliness, nothing to taint or destroy, nothing to cause disease or death.

Let physicians and nurses draw from the things of nature, lessons teaching of God. Let them point the patients to Him whose hand has made the lofty trees, the grass, and the flowers, encouraging them to see in every bud and flower an expression of His love for His children. He who cares for the birds and the flowers will care for the beings formed in His own image.

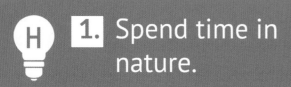

H 1. Spend time in nature.

Out of doors, amid the things that God has made, breathing the fresh, health-giving air, the sick can best be told of the new life in Christ. Here God's word can be read. Here the light of Christ's righteousness can shine into hearts darkened by sin.

Men and women in need of physical and spiritual healing are to be thus brought into contact with those whose words and acts will draw them to Christ. They are to be brought under the influence of the great Medical Missionary, who can heal both soul and body. They are to hear

the story of the Savior's love, of the pardon freely provided for all who come to Him confessing their sins.

Under such influences as these, many suffering ones will be guided into the way of life. Angels of heaven cooperate with human instrumentalities in bringing encouragement and hope and joy and peace to the hearts of the sick and suffering. Under such conditions the sick are doubly blessed, and many find health. The feeble step recovers its elasticity. The eye regains its brightness. The hopeless become hopeful. The once despondent face wears an expression of joy. The complaining tones of the voice give place to tones of cheerfulness and contentment.

As physical health is regained, men and women are better able to exercise that faith in Christ which secures the health of the soul. In the consciousness of sins forgiven there is inexpressible peace and joy and rest. The clouded hope of the Christian is brightened. The words express the belief, "God is our refuge and strength, a very present help in trouble." "Yea, though I walk through the valley of the shadow of death, I will fear no evil: for Thou art with me; Thy rod and Thy staff they comfort me." "He giveth power to the faint; and to them that have no might He increaseth strength." Psalm 46:1; 23:4; Isaiah 40:29. ~ The Ministry of Healing, pages 261-267.

Our surroundings affect us more than we think. People tend to be more at peace where there is nature. Smog, traffic, and the city life can wear us out more than we think. It is advisable that we live in an area with clean air, beautiful, sunny weather, and in a safe neighborhood. If that is not possible, it would be beneficial for us to go and spend time in nature as much and as frequently as possible.

Not only does the area or the neighborhood in which we live in affect us, but how we live in our homes affects our well-being as well. A clean home is not only pleasant to live in but it is also very important for good health.

In the teaching that God gave to Israel, the preservation of health received careful attention. The people who had come from slavery with the uncleanly and unhealthful habits which it engenders were subjected to the strictest training in the wilderness before entering Canaan. Health principles were taught and sanitary laws enforced.

Not only in their religious service, but in all the affairs of daily life they observed the distinction between clean and unclean. All who came in contact with contagious or contaminating diseases were isolated from the encampment, and they were not permitted to return without thorough cleansing of both the person and the clothing. In

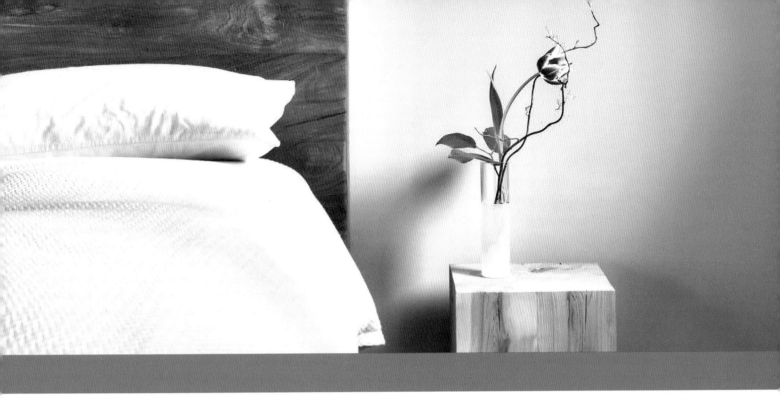

the case of one afflicted with a contaminating disease, the direction was given:

"Every bed, whereon he lieth, . . . is unclean: and everything, whereon he sitteth, shall be unclean. And whosoever toucheth his bed shall wash his clothes, and bathe himself in water, and be unclean until the even. And he that sitteth on anything whereon he sat . . . shall wash his clothes, and bathe himself in water, and be unclean until the even. And he that toucheth the flesh of him . . . shall wash his clothes, and bathe himself in water, and be unclean until the even. . . . And whosoever toucheth anything that was under him shall be unclean until the even: and he that beareth any of those things shall wash his clothes, and bathe himself in water, and be unclean until the even. And whomsoever he toucheth . . . and hath not rinsed his hands in water, he shall wash his clothes, and bathe himself in water, and be unclean until the even. And the vessel of earth, that he toucheth, . . . shall be broken: and every vessel of wood shall be rinsed in water." Leviticus 15:4-12.

The law concerning leprosy is also an illustration of the thoroughness with which these regulations were to be enforced:

"All the days wherein the plague shall be in him [the leper] he shall be defiled; he is unclean: he shall dwell alone; without the camp shall his habitation be. The garment also that the plague of leprosy is in, whether it be a woolen garment, or a linen garment; whether it be in the warp, or woof; of linen, or of woolen; whether in a skin, or in anything made of skin; . . . the priest shall look upon the plague: . . . if the plague be spread in the garment, either in the warp, or in the woof, or in a skin, or in any work that is made of skin; the plague is a fretting leprosy; it is unclean. He shall therefore burn that garment, whether warp or woof, in woolen or in linen, or anything of skin, wherein the plague is: for it is a fretting leprosy; it shall be burnt in the fire." Leviticus 13:46-52.

So, too, if a house gave evidence of conditions that rendered it unsafe for habitation, it was destroyed. The priest was to "break down the house, the stones of it, and the timber thereof, and all the mortar of the house; and he shall carry them forth out of the city into an unclean place. Moreover he that goeth into the house all the while that it is shut up shall be unclean until the even. And he that lieth in the house shall wash his clothes; and he that eateth in the house shall wash his clothes." Leviticus 14:45-47.

The necessity of personal cleanliness was taught in the most impressive manner. Before gathering at Mount Sinai to listen to the proclamation of the law by the voice of God, the people were required to wash both their persons and their clothing. This direction was enforced on pain of death. No impurity was to be tolerated in the presence of God.

During their stay in the wilderness the Israelites were almost continually in the open air, where impurities would have a less harmful effect than upon the dwellers in close houses. But the strictest regard to cleanliness was required both within and without their tents. No refuse was allowed to remain within or about the encampment. The Lord said:

"The Lord thy God walketh in the midst of thy camp, to deliver thee, and to give up thine enemies before thee; therefore shall thy camp be holy." *Deuteronomy 23:14.* ~ *The Ministry of Healing,* pages 277-280.

Scrupulous cleanliness is essential to both physical and mental health. . . . *Every form of uncleanliness tends to disease. Death-producing germs abound in dark, neglected corners, in decaying refuse, in dampness and mold and must. No waste vegetables or heaps of fallen leaves should be allowed to remain near the house to decay and poison the air. Nothing unclean or decaying should be tolerated within the home.* ~ *The Ministry of Healing,* page 276.

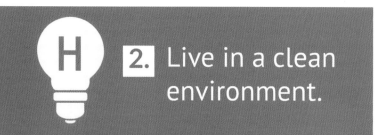

H 2. Live in a clean environment.

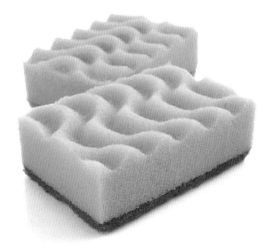

Perfect cleanliness, plenty of sunlight, careful attention to sanitation in every detail of the home life, are essential to freedom from disease and to the cheerfulness and vigor of all who live in the home.
~ *The Ministry of Healing,* page 276.

Six of the Most Surprisingly Dirty Places in Your Home:

1) "Food particles from plates left to soak or rinsed from dishes on their way to the dishwasher can serve as a breeding ground for illness-causing bacteria, including E. coli and salmonella. They can get on your hands or spread to foods." [5]

2) Many experts would agree that the toilet bowl could be cleaner than the average kitchen sink!

3) The solution: "To sanitize your sink and prevent the spread of bacteria, wash it with a solution of bleach and water once a day and then let the solution run down the drain. Remember to remove the drain plug and clean it, too! Then wash your hands." [6]

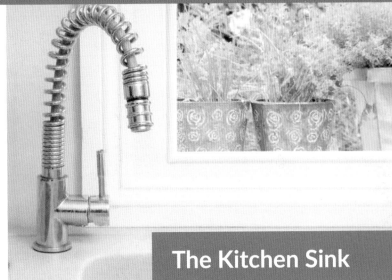

The Kitchen Sink

Your Tooth Brush

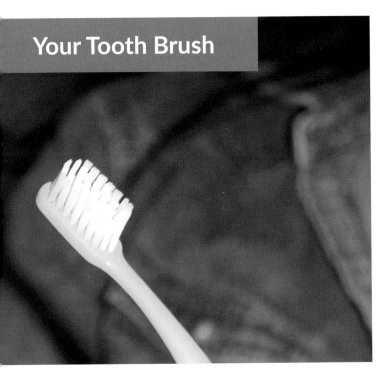

1) "You put it in your mouth twice a day, but do you ever think of all the germs lurking on it? You rinse it off after using it and put it away damp. If the germs from your own mouth weren't enough to contaminate your toothbrush, the germs from your toilet certainly are. Research in the 1970s by Charles P. Gerba, PhD, of the University of Arizona Department of Soil, Water and Environmental Science, found that flushing the toilet sends a spray of bacteria- and virus-contaminated water droplets into air. These germs, he found, can float around in the bathroom for at least two hours after each flush before landing on surfaces—including your toothbrush." [7]

2) The solution: Place your toothbrush where it can air out and dry between uses—"but not too close to the toilet. Also, replace your toothbrush often, particularly after you've been sick, and close your toilet lid before flushing." [8]

1) "The place where you clean yourself is not so clean itself. A recent study found staphylococcus bacteria in 26% of the tubs tested." [9]

2) The solution: "Experts recommend cleaning and disinfecting your tub with bleach or bathroom cleaner after bathing, then dry with a clean towel." [10]

The Bathtub

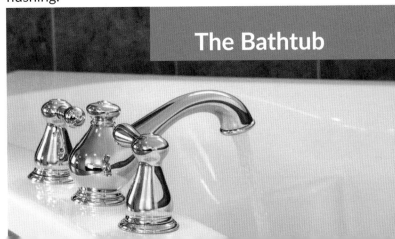

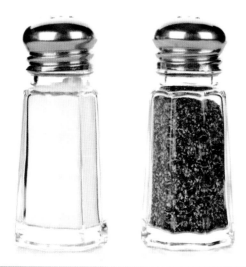

1) In a 2008 study by researchers at the University of Virginia, "the researchers asked 30 adults who were beginning to show signs of a cold, to name 10 places they'd touched in their homes over the previous 18 hours. The researchers then tested those areas for cold viruses. The tests found viruses on 41% of the surfaces tested, and every one of the salt and pepper shakers tested were positive for cold viruses." [11] Yikes!

2) The solution: "When you wipe the kitchen table after eating, wipe off the salt and pepper shaker too." [12]

Your Salt and Pepper Shaker

1.) "A University of Virginia study of cold viruses on household surfaces showed the remote control's surface is among the germiest! Researchers found that half of the remote controls tested were positive for cold viruses." [13]

2) The solution: Wipe off your remote with a bleach or alcohol wipe. "Aside from that, regular hand-washing is the best way to protect yourself against these germs." [14]

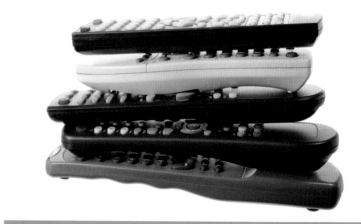

The TV Remote

Your Computer Keyboard

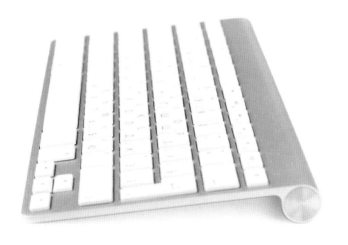

1) "If you eat at your computer, sneeze on your keyboard, or sit down to surf the Internet without first washing your hands, your computer keyboard could be a health hazard. In a recent study by a British consumer group, researchers swabbed keyboards for germs and found a host of potentially harmful bacteria, including E. coli and staph. Four of 33 sampled keyboards had enough germs to be considered health hazards. One had levels of germs five times higher than that found on a toilet seat." [15]

2) The solution: "Wash your hands before and after using your computer. If you must eat at your desk, don't drop crumbs into your keyboard. To clean your keyboard, gently shake out the crumbs or vacuum it. Wiping the keys with alcohol or bleach wipes can help, but nothing too wet. And don't forget to wipe the mouse." [16]

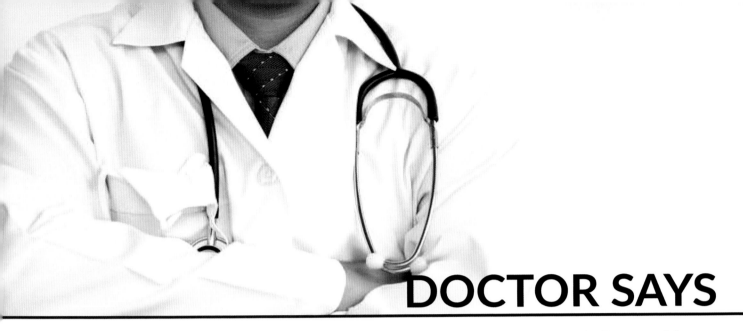

DOCTOR SAYS

People who live in a healthy community tend to be healthier. We are influenced by our friends, workplace, family, church, school etc. It is easier to be healthy around people that are healthy. Choose to spend time with positive influences and close to nature.

- Spend time in nature.
- Live in a clean area.
- Join an exercise group.
- Join some sort of health club.
- Associate yourself with others who want to achieve the same goal of good health as you do.

FRESH AIR & SUNLIGHT

To afford the most favorable conditions for recovery, the room that the sick person occupies should be large, sunny, and cheerfully decorated, with thorough ventilation. . . . Every possible effort should be made to arrange the sickroom so that a current of fresh air can pass through it night and day. ~ The Ministry of Healing, page 220.

Earlier we mentioned about the importance of spending time in nature and living in a clean environment. One reason why spending time outdoors in nature can benefit our health is because of the fresh air and the sunlight that we get. Like in Henry and Anna's situation, it is becoming a luxury for many Americans to get a daily dose of fresh air and sunshine. Read on to learn why this may be more than a luxury, but a necessity for good health.

In order to have good blood, we must breathe well. Full, deep breaths of pure air, which fill the lungs with oxygen, purify the blood. They impart to it a bright color and send it, a life-giving current, to every part of the body. A good respiration soothes the nerves; it stimulates the appetite and improves the digestion; and it induces sound, refreshing sleep.

The lungs should be allowed the greatest freedom possible. Their capacity is developed by free action; it diminishes if they are cramped and compressed. Hence the ill effects of the practice so common, especially in sedentary pursuits, of stooping at one's work. In this position it is impossible to breathe deeply. Superficial breathing soon becomes a habit, and the lungs lose their power to expand.

Thus an insufficient supply of oxygen is received. The blood moves sluggishly. The waste, poisonous matter, which should be thrown off in the exhalations from the lungs, is retained, and the blood becomes impure. Not only the lungs, but the stomach, liver, and brain are affected. The skin becomes sallow, digestion is slowed; the heart is depressed; the brain is clouded; the thoughts are confused; gloom settles upon the spirits; the whole system becomes depressed and inactive, and peculiarly susceptible to disease. ~ The Ministry of Healing, pages 272, 273.

Our bodies need oxygen from the air around us to function. The lungs absorb the oxygen from the air we inhale, the oxygen is then given to the red blood cells, and the blood carries the oxygen to the various organs such as the brain, liver, and the heart. The blood also carries away the waste and the carbon dioxide from these organs. Without oxygen the cells in our bodies start being unable to function and eventually die. [1,2]

That is why we are programmed to breathe automatically. We breathe without consciously needing to tell ourselves to. But, every now and then, we need to remind ourselves to sit up straight or stand tall and breathe deeply. Although a healthy person may take breathing naturally and unconsciously for granted, it can be very refreshing and rejuvenating to take a deep breath of clean, fresh air. Here are some tips: [3]

1. Find a relatively peaceful place with clean, fresh air. Preferably the outdoors amidst greenery.
2. Place one hand on your abdomen, just below your ribs. Place the other hand on your chest. Take a regular breath.
3. Now take a slow, deep breath. Breathe in slowly through your nose. Pay attention as your abdomen expands under your hand.
4. Holding your breath, pause for a second or two.
5. Slowly breathe out through your mouth. Pay attention as the hand on your abdomen goes in with the breath.
6. Repeat several times.

The lungs are constantly throwing off impurities, and they need to be constantly supplied with fresh air. Impure air does not afford the necessary supply of oxygen, and the blood passes to the brain and other organs without being vitalized. Hence the necessity of thorough ventilation. To live in close, ill-ventilated rooms, where the air is dead and depleted, weakens the entire system. It becomes peculiarly sensitive to the influence of cold, and a slight exposure induces disease. It is close confinement indoors that makes many people, especially some women, pale and feeble. They breathe the same air over and over until it becomes laden with poisonous matter thrown off through the lungs and pores, and impurities are thus conveyed back to the blood.

In the construction of buildings, whether for public purposes or as dwellings, care should be taken to provide for good ventilation and plenty of sunlight. Churches and schoolrooms are often faulty in this respect. Neglect of proper ventilation is responsible for much of the drowsiness and dullness that destroy the

SOME POTENTIAL BENEFITS OF DEEP BREATHING [4]
- RELIEVES STRESS
- RELAXES TENSE MUSCLES
- LOWERS BLOOD PRESSURE

effect of many a sermon and make the teacher's work difficult and ineffective. ~ The Ministry of Healing, page 274.

Have you ever sat in a sermon, lecture, or class and started to feel sleepy? Sometimes, the presenter may be boring or you have not had enough sleep lately. But other times you've had plenty of good rest, the presenter is really interesting, and still you start to feel so slow and drowsy. Have you ever wondered why that is? There is a possible explanation for that. Often, when we are listening to someone speak, there are many other people in the room listening. We are seated or standing close to each other and the air around us doesn't feel so fresh anymore.

As mentioned earlier, we need oxygen to survive. When we inhale, we are breathing in to try to get that oxygen to our various organs. When we exhale, we are breathing out the carbon dioxide that the organs are

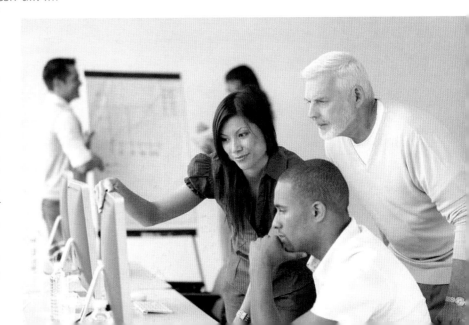

trying to get rid of. When we are in a crowded room with no ventilation, we begin to breathe in each other's exhaled air. The air starts being filled with more and more carbon dioxide and less and less oxygen. The brain needs a lot of oxygen. [5] Although it is only about

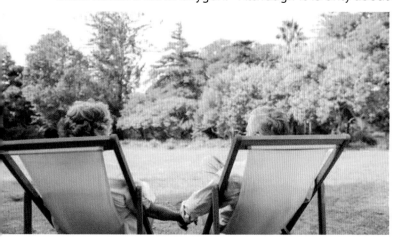

2 percent of the entire body weight, it receives about 15 percent to 20 percent of the body's blood supply to meet its oxygen needs. Without the fresh supply of blood with oxygen, the brain cells will begin to die. [6]

H

1. Open the windows or get good ventilation when sitting in a crowded classroom or a packed meeting room.

2. Leave the window open a crack, or get good ventilation while sleeping.

A study published in the Environmental Health Perspectives suggests that breathing in the carbon dioxide exhaled by those around you could cause you to think more slowly. [7] This study indicated that people's decision making performance declined in various activities that they undertook. For this reason proper ventilation could help improve your learning experience. Not only could it help in classroom and meeting room settings, but also while you sleep. Even if we sleep by ourselves, when a room is small and enclosed with windows and doors completely shut, we may start breathing in more of our exhaled carbon dioxide than the much needed fresh oxygen.

In the building of houses it is especially important to secure thorough ventilation and plenty of sunlight. Let there be a current of air and an abundance of light in every room in the house. Sleeping rooms should be so arranged as to have a free circulation of air day and night. No room is fit to be occupied as a sleeping room unless it can be thrown open daily to the air and sunshine. In most countries bedrooms need to be supplied with conveniences for heating, that they may be thoroughly warmed and dried in cold or wet weather.

In building, many make careful provision for their plants and flowers. The greenhouse or window devoted to their use is warm and sunny; for without warmth, air, and sunshine, plants would not live and flourish. If these conditions are necessary to the life of plants, how much more necessary are they for our own health and that of our families and guests!

If we would have our homes be the place where health and happiness abide, we must give free entrance to heaven's life-giving agencies. Dispense with heavy curtains, open the windows and the blinds, allow no vines, however beautiful, to shade the windows, and permit no trees to stand so near the house as to shut out the sunshine. The sunlight may fade the drapery and the carpets, and tarnish the picture frames; but it will bring a healthy glow to the cheeks of the children.

Those who have the elderly to provide for should remember that these especially need warm, comfortable rooms. Vigor declines as years advance, leaving less vitality with which to resist unhealthful influences; hence the greater importance for the elderly to have plenty of sunlight, and fresh, pure air. ~ The Ministry of Healing, pages 274, 275.

THE BENEFITS OF MODERATE SUNLIGHT EXPOSURE:

1 Promotes Vitamin D Production
Vitamin D is necessary for many things such as healthy bone formation, proper immune function, cell growth, nerve and muscle function, and reducing inflammation. Research also suggests that a proper amount of Vitamin D could play a role in preventing and treating various other diseases such as type 1 and 2 diabetes, hypertension, glucose intolerance, and even multiple sclerosis. [8]

2 Better Mood
Have you ever thought why we commonly refer to somebody's good mood as a "sunny disposition?" Or why do we associate the lack of sun-

shine with sadness or gloominess? There may be a reason for this. There is a type of depression called Seasonal Affective Disorder that affects some people during the winter months when they don't get enough sunlight.[9] Unsurprisingly, experts now believe that the sunlight has widespread mood-elevating effects on us. I mean, who doesn't like relaxing on a warm, sunny day?

3 Cancer Prevention

Although too much sunshine can lead to skin cancers, studies have shown that other cancers and infectious diseases could result from too little sunshine.[10] The risk of dying from breast, ovarian, colon, pancreatic, prostate, and other cancers was higher in those who got too little sunshine.[11]

4 Autoimmune Conditions

According to a report published in the Environmental Health Perspectives, exposure to UV radiation appears to suppress an overactive immune system. "This could explain why exposure to UV rays may help with autoimmune diseases like psoriasis and lupus; one recent study also suggests it might help alleviate asthma."[12]

5 Better Sleep

Natural sunlight can balance out the production of melatonin, a hormone produced at night that makes you drowsy. "This can help you maintain a normal circadian rhythm, so you're more likely to feel tired at bedtime when it's dark outside. Going outside for fifteen minutes at the same time each day, preferably in the morning, gives your body a clear signal that it's no longer night."[13] Getting proper amounts of natural sunlight can especially help the elderly, since melatonin production is known to decrease as we age.[14]

6 Joint Pain

A Harvard study indicated that exposure to UVB rays from sunlight is associated with the decreased risk of developing rheumatoid arthritis, a painful autoimmune disease in which the lining of the joints swells up due to the body mistakenly attacking its own tissues. Women with the highest UVB exposure had a 21 percent decreased risk of developing this disease in comparison to those who had the lowest.[15,16]

H **3.** Go outside, get some fresh air and sunshine! But, not too much. Depending on the fairness of your skin, ten to twenty minutes a day seems to be the average recommended amount.

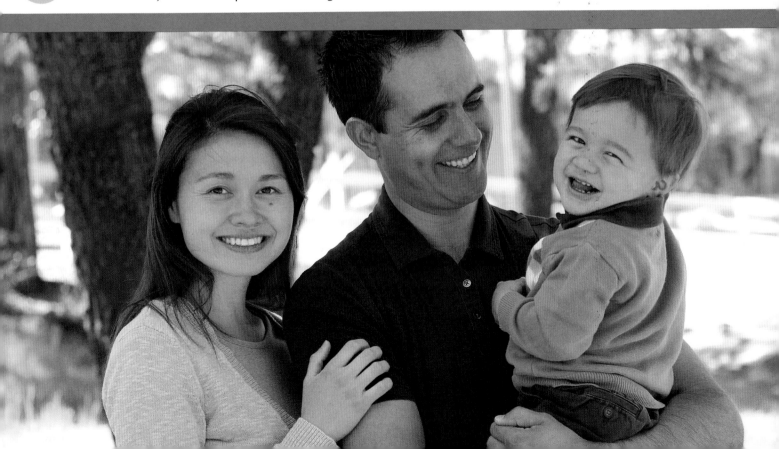

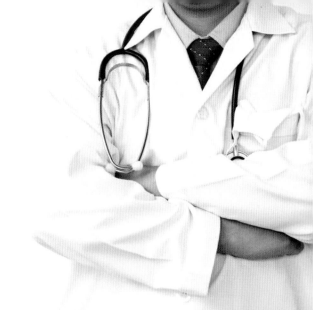

7 Brain Function

According to a study published in the Journal of the American Medical Association, "Elderly Alzheimer's patients exposed to bright lighting during the day—from 9 a.m. to 6 p.m.—got better scores on a mental exam, had fewer symptoms of depression, and lost less function than did those exposed to dim daytime lighting."[17] The researchers attributed the improvement to a more regular circadian rhythm due to exposure to sunlight. [18]

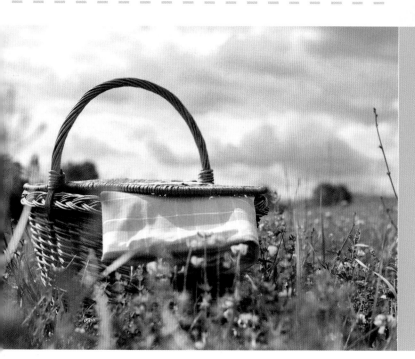

DOCTOR SAYS

Fresh air and proper amounts of sunlight are very important for your health. Especially in Vitamin D synthesis and proper melatonin production, sunlight plays a major role. Here are some fun, easy ways to get some fresh air and sunlight:

- Have a picnic.
- Eat lunch outside.
- If it is close by, walk to where you buy lunch.
- Have family time on the patio or in the backyard instead of in front of the TV.
- Take a short walk after meals.

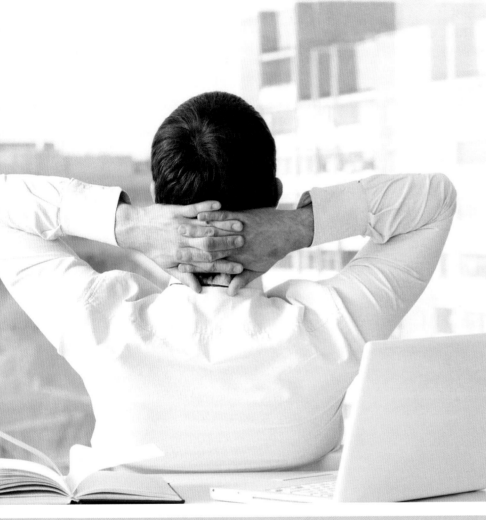

Habit #7

HEALTHY
BALANCE

Some make themselves sick by overwork. For these, rest, freedom from care, and a moderate diet, are essential to restoration of health. To those who are brain weary and nervous because of continual labor and close confinement, a visit to the country, where they can live a simple, carefree life, coming in close contact with the things of nature, will be most helpful. Roaming through the fields and the woods, picking the flowers, listening to the songs of the birds, will do far more than any other agency toward their recovery. ~The Ministry of Healing, pages 236, 237.

Many Americans live unbalanced lives. For example, Henry travels about forty-five minutes in traffic to get to his office. He sits in front of a computer most of the day with an earpiece, getting up occasionally for some coffee or to go to a meeting. Anna also travels through traffic for about thirty-five minutes to her work as the hospital front desk receptionist. She also remains indoors and is sedentary for most of the day.

They both don't get any sunlight or fresh air during the weekdays with the exception of walking between their office doors and parked cars. Because they are trying to pay off their credit card debt, they have been working every other weekend and also some holidays.

Henry and Anna have one 16-year-old son left at home, but they hardly get to spend time with him. They used to take occasional camping trips and other family vacations, but once their other two children moved out, fun family vacations disappeared and even their family leisure time diminished. Now their family pastime is watching TV shows after dinner, lethargically sprawled out on their big, fluffy couch with a container of bite-size brownies, usually without their youngest son.

Working hard, making an honest living, and providing for your family are all very good things. But getting exercise, spending time with your children, and getting rest and rejuvenation from nature and from God are also very good things. You see, it is a balance of these many very good things that gives us a healthy life.

Disease never comes without a cause. The way is prepared, and disease invited, by disregard of the laws of health.* Many suffer in consequence of the transgression of their parents. While they are not responsible for what their parents have done, it is nevertheless their duty to ascertain what are and what are not violations of the laws of health. They should avoid the wrong habits of their parents and, by correct living, place themselves in better conditions.

The greater number, however, suffer because of their own wrong course of action. They disregard the principles of health by their habits of eating, drinking, dressing, and working. Their transgression of nature's laws produces the sure result; and when sickness comes upon them, many do not credit their suffering to the true cause, but murmur against God because of their afflictions. But God is not responsible for the suffering that follows disregard of natural law.

God has endowed us with a certain amount of vital force. He has also formed us with organs suited to maintain the various functions of life, and He designs that these organs shall work together in harmony. If we carefully preserve the life force, and keep the delicate mechanism of the body in order, the result is health; but if the vital force is too rapidly exhausted, the nervous system borrows power for present use from its resources of strength, and when one organ is injured, all are affected. Nature bears much abuse without apparent resistance; she then arouses and makes a determined effort to remove the effects of the ill-treatment she has suffered. Her effort to correct these conditions is often manifest in fever and various other forms of sickness.

When the abuse of health is carried so far that sickness results, the sufferer can often do for himself what no one else can do for him. The first thing to be done is to ascertain the true character of the sickness and then go to work intelligently to remove the cause. If the harmonious working of the system has become unbalanced by overwork, overeating, or other irregularities, do not endeavor to adjust the difficulties by adding a burden of poisonous medicines.

Intemperate eating is often the cause of sickness, and what nature most needs is to be relieved of the undue burden that has been placed upon her. In many cases of sickness, the very best remedy is for the patient to fast for a meal or two, that the overworked organs of digestion may have an opportunity to rest. A fruit diet for a few days has often brought great relief to brain workers. Many times a short period of entire abstinence from food, followed by simple, moderate eating, has led to recovery through nature's own recuperative effort. A careful, restrained diet for a month or two would convince many sufferers that the path of self-denial is the path to health.

Some make themselves sick by overwork. For these, rest, freedom from care, and a moderate diet, are essential to restoration of health. To those who are brain weary and nervous because of continual labor and close confinement, a visit to the country, where they can live a simple, carefree life, coming in close contact with the things of nature, will be most helpful. Roaming through the fields and the woods, picking the flowers, listening to the songs of the birds, will do far more than any other agency toward their recovery. ~ The Ministry of Healing, pages 234-237.

> The first thing to be done is to ascertain the true character of the sickness and then go to work intelligently to remove the cause.

---

*We may not understand the exact cause of some diseases, but all diseases have causes. The cause may not even be your fault, or your parents' fault or anybody else's fault. The diseased person may have lived a very healthy, principled life but may still get sick. Often times there are diseases that develop of which we do not know the cause. In fact, most people will experience major sickness in their lives or in the lives of their loved ones.

The long-living Seventh-day Adventists help keep a healthy balance in their busy lives by devoting one whole day, one 24-hour period, to refresh and rejuvenate. They keep what is called the Sabbath, as mentioned throughout the Bible.** They reserve the time from Friday night to Saturday night to spend with their families and friends, serving the community, and seeking spiritual and physical rejuvenation. During this time, they typically do not go to work or answer business calls or emails, but they let themselves be carefree from the daily stresses of life. This day is a special day that these long-living Seventh-day Adventists look forward to throughout the week and can be considered as a weekly mini-vacation.

**Genesis 2:2-3; Exodus 20:8-11; Deuteronomy 5:12-15; Mark 2:27, 28

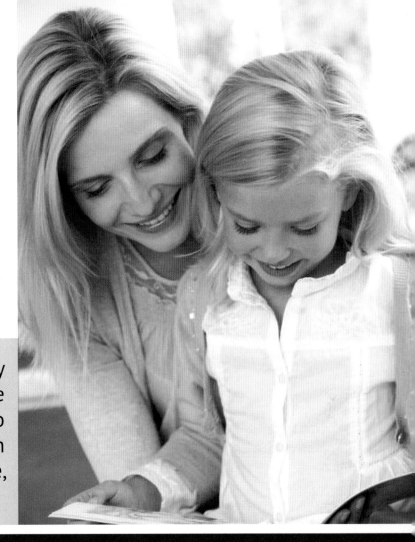

1. Take a weekly one-day vacation. Reserve one whole day every week to pause and unwind from the daily stresses of life, work, and/or school.

Some fun ideas to refresh and rejuvenate on this day:

- Rest
- Spend time in nature
- Hike
- Picnic
- Sing and pray
- Worship and fellowship
- Bible study
- Volunteer ministries
- Outreach to the community

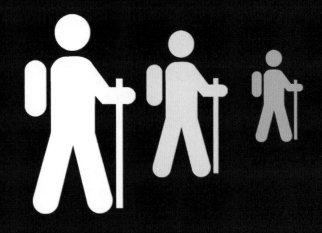

One of the major things that many Americans have difficulty managing is the balance between their work and personal life. There are numerous articles and other publications on this subject. Here are some ideas and tips that are mentioned in various articles.[1,2]

1. Schedule down time into your day. Many work longer than they wish and spend less time where they really want to spend it. We don't think twice about scheduling business meetings into our busy days or lunch with a potential client. Why not schedule family dinners or playtime with your children into your routine?

2. Cut out the things that don't add value to your life. How often do we waste precious time on things that don't really matter or benefit us in our lives? Television, Internet, video games—is this really the way that we want to pass our sunny weekends? Why not spend time with your family and loved ones instead? Play outside with your kids, go on a picnic, make memories with the people that matter most to you. These things can be done if we cut off the things that suck out our valuable time and energy.

3. Choose wisely who to spend time and energy with. Not only do we spend time on things and entertainment that don't edify us, but sometimes there are people in our lives that can negatively influence us—the people around us who only want to gossip, speak negatively, or constantly vent for hours on end with no intention of solving their issues. Limit your time with these kinds of people. Avoid them if you can. Choose to spend time with people who bring the best out of you.

4. Rethink your tasks and errands. Are there things that you can do differently or delegate to free you up to do the things that only you can do? Do you really have to wash those dishes, or can the dishwasher handle that? Can you hire the kid next door to mow the lawn for you? Some people like to get their groceries online and delivered to their doorstep; with just a few extra dollars they can free up a few extra hours.

How about exchanging services with your friends or neighbors? If you enjoy cooking, offer to cook meals for them in exchange for some other chore that you don't enjoy as much. How about taking turns with the neighbor mom, watching each others' kids, freeing up time to take care of errands and chores that are done more quickly without the kids?

5. Make time for yourself. Last but not least, make sure you take some time to rejuvenate and refresh. You will be able to perform your job more effectively and be a better companion to those around you. Take time to enjoy your hobby, read a good book, pray, reflect, catch up with friends, etc.

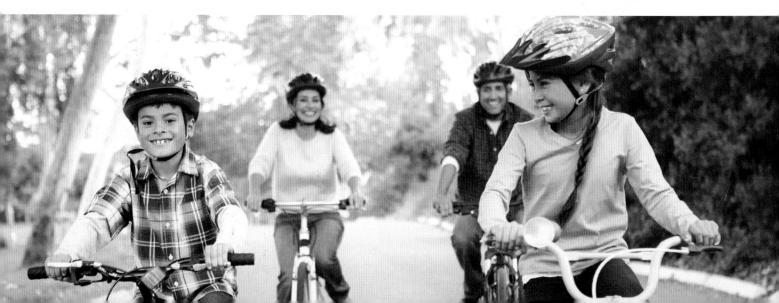

Right now this is what Anna's typical weekday looks like:

6:00 am Alarm starts going off every five minutes.

6:40 am Finally gets out of bed in a rush

6:45 am Hops in the shower and gets ready for the day: hair, dress, make-up, brushes teeth

7:45 am Hurriedly comes into the kitchen to turn the coffee maker on, grabs her socks, looks in the fridge and mentally calculates what she needs to buy, speaks a few words to Henry and their son, sometimes eats breakfast when she has the time

7:55 am Grabs her coffee and rushes out of the garage for work hoping there is not as much traffic as usual

8:30 am Pulls into the hospital parking lot wishing she had left the house just five minutes earlier

8:36 am Clocks in for work, hoping nobody noticed that she had come in a little late, as usual. Sits in front of the computer for most of the morning, occasionally getting up to get some coffee and snacks from the break room

12:30 pm Eats lunch

1:00 pm Sits in front of the computer for most of the afternoon and gets up occasionally for coffee and snacks or to help a confused person navigate to the proper place

5:10 pm Heads outside to her car in the parking lot

5:30 pm Stops by the supermarket to pick up groceries or one of the restaurants to pick up dinner

6:25 pm Arrives home

6:40 pm Turns the TV on and fixes dinner or heats up the take-out

7:15 pm Eats dinner with Henry and sometimes their son with the TV turned on

7:50 pm Cleans kitchen

8:30 pm Lounges around, eats some dessert while watching TV

11:30 pm Is exhausted and goes to bed but tosses and turns for some time

12:30 am Finally falls asleep

Henry's typical weekday and some weekends when he and Anna work:

6:00 am Anna's alarm starts going off every five minutes.

6:40 am Nudges Anna to get out of bed and turn off the alarm

7:00 am Drowsily gets out of bed

7:10 am Showers and gets ready for the day

7:40 am Turns the news on

7:50 am Checks how his favorite sports team is doing and exchanges a few words with Anna and their son

8:10 am Grabs a cereal bar and orange-flavored drink from the kitchen to eat and drink while stuck in traffic. Drives out of the garage for work

9:00 am Clocks in for work. Remains seated in front of his desk for most of the day. Occasionally gets up to get coffee and snacks

12:30 pm Eats lunch

1:30 pm Works in front of his desk for most of the afternoon. Gets up a couple of times to go to meetings or to get some coffee and snacks

6:00 pm Leaves work

7:00 pm Arrives home and changes into comfortable clothing

7:15 pm Eats dinner with Anna and sometimes their son

8:00 pm Watches TV and has some snacks and soda

11:20 pm Starts heading to bed

11:45 pm Falls asleep

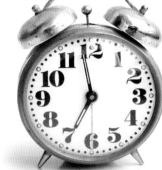

Their day-to-day schedule plus every other weekend look like this. What kinds of changes could Henry and Anna make? Perhaps more exercise and less TV? More interaction with each other and their son? A healthful breakfast instead of coffee and snacks? Write out here what kinds of changes you would make if you were Henry or Anna.

_____

_____

_____

_____

_____

_____

_____

Take a moment to think and evaluate your life. Are you content with where you spend your time? Are you happy and excited about the direction that your life is heading in?

Changes in your life begin by the choices you make on a day-to-day basis. Take a record of how you spend your day and evaluate if you are happy with how the day was spent.

Are you happy with how your day was spent? Are there any changes that you would like to make? If so, write out what your day could look like with the improved changes.

Time		Time	
4:00 am	_____	4:00 am	_____
5:00 am	_____	5:00 am	_____
6:00 am	_____	6:00 am	_____
7:00 am	_____	7:00 am	_____
8:00 am	_____	8:00 am	_____
9:00 am	_____	9:00 am	_____
10:00 am	_____	10:00 am	_____
11:00 am	_____	11:00 am	_____
12:00 pm	_____	12:00 pm	_____
1:00 pm	_____	1:00 pm	_____
2:00 pm	_____	2:00 pm	_____
3:00 pm	_____	3:00 pm	_____
4:00 pm	_____	4:00 pm	_____
5:00 pm	_____	5:00 pm	_____
6:00 pm	_____	6:00 pm	_____
7:00 pm	_____	7:00 pm	_____
8:00 pm	_____	8:00 pm	_____
9:00 pm	_____	9:00 pm	_____
10:00 pm	_____	10:00 pm	_____
11:00 pm	_____	11:00 pm	_____
12:00 am	_____	12:00 am	_____
1:00 am	_____	1:00 am	_____
2:00 am	_____	2:00 am	_____
3:00 am	_____	3:00 am	_____

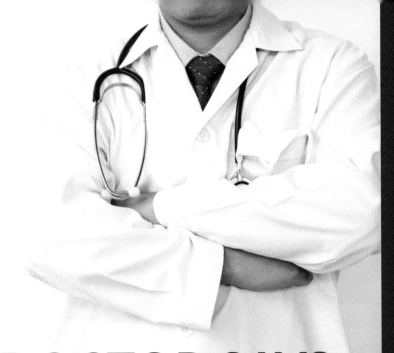

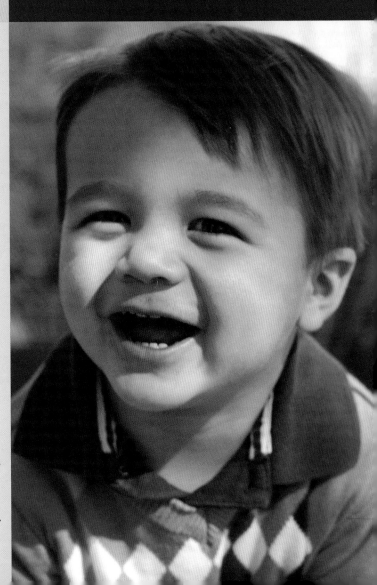

God has endowed us with a certain amount of vital force. He has also formed us with organs suited to maintain the various functions of life, and He designs that these organs shall work together in harmony. If we carefully preserve the life force, and keep the delicate mechanism of the body in order, the result is health.

DOCTOR SAYS

This wise man said it best:

"To everything there is a season, and a time to every purpose under the heaven:
A time to be born, and a time to die; a time to plant, and a time to pluck up that which is planted;
A time to kill, and a time to heal; a time to break down, and a time to build up;
A time to weep, and a time to laugh; a time to mourn, and a time to dance;
A time to cast away stones, and a time to gather stones together; a time to embrace, and a time to refrain from embracing;
A time to get, and a time to lose; a time to keep, and a time to cast away;
A time to love, and a time to hate; a time of war, and a time of peace.
He hath made everything beautiful in his time...
And also that every man should eat and drink, and enjoy the good of all his labour, it is the gift of God."
- Ecclesiastes 3:1-8, 11, 13.

There is a time for everything. Everyone has 24 hours in a day. Balance those 24 hours appropriately. Take time to work hard and enjoy the rewards of your work afterward. Make time for the people that matter most to you. Make time for God. Take time to take care of yourself and enjoy life. You will be healthier and happier.

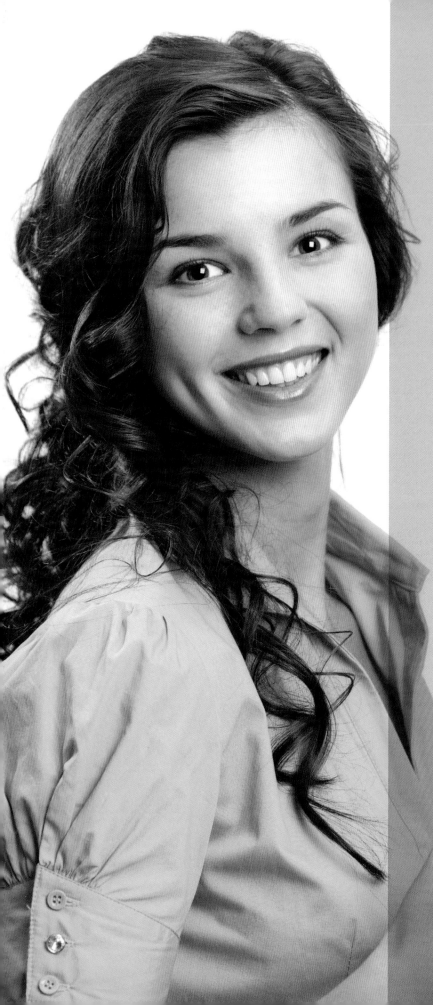

EAT TO LIVE

Our bodies are built up from the food we eat. ~The Ministry of Healing, page 295.

O ur bodies are built up from the food we eat. There is a constant breaking down of the tissues of the body; every movement of every organ involves waste, and this waste is repaired from our food. Each organ of the body requires its share of nutrition. The brain must be supplied with its portion; the bones, muscles, and nerves demand theirs. It is a wonderful process that transforms the food into blood and uses this blood to build up the varied parts of the body; but this process is going on continually, supplying with life and strength each nerve, muscle, and tissue.

Those foods should be chosen that best supply the elements needed for building up the body. In this choice, appetite is not a safe guide. Through wrong habits of eating, the appetite has become perverted. Often it demands food that impairs health and causes weakness instead of strength. We cannot safely be guided by the customs of society. The disease and suffering that everywhere prevail are largely due to popular errors in regard to diet.

In order to know what are the best foods, we must study God's original plan for man's diet. He who created man and who understands his needs appointed Adam his food. "Behold," He said, "I have given you every herb yielding seed, . . . and every tree, in which is the fruit of a tree yielding seed; to you it shall be for food." Genesis 1:29, A.R.V. Upon leaving Eden to gain his livelihood by tilling the earth under the curse of sin, man received permission to eat also "the herb of the field." Genesis 3:18.

Grains, fruits, nuts, and vegetables constitute the diet chosen for us by our Creator. These foods, prepared in as simple and natural a manner as possible, are the most healthful and nourishing. They impart a strength, a power of endurance, and a vigor of intellect that are not afforded by a more complex and stimulating diet.

But not all foods wholesome in themselves are equally suited to our needs under all circumstances. Care should be taken in the selection of food. Our diet should be suited to the season, to the climate in which we live, and to the occupation we follow. Some foods that are adapted for use at one season or in one climate are not suited to another. So there are different foods best suited for persons in different occupations. Often food that can be used with benefit by those engaged in hard physical labor is unsuitable for persons of sedentary pursuits or intense mental application. God has given us an ample variety of healthful foods, and each person should choose from it the things that experience and sound judgment prove to be best suited to his own necessities.

Nuts and nut foods are coming largely into use to take the place of flesh meats. With nuts may be combined grains, fruits, and some roots, to make foods that are healthful and nourishing. Care should be taken, however, not to use too large a proportion of nuts. Those who realize ill effects from the use of nut foods may find the difficulty removed by following this precaution. It should be remembered, too, that some nuts are not so wholesome as others. Almonds are preferable to peanuts, but peanuts in limited quantities, used in connection with grains, are nourishing and digestible.

When properly prepared, olives, like nuts, supply the place of butter and flesh meats. The oil, as eaten in the olive, is far preferable to animal oil or fat.

Persons who have accustomed themselves to a rich, highly stimulating diet have an unnatural taste, and they cannot at once relish food that is plain and simple. It will take time for the taste to become natural and for the stomach to recover from the abuse it has suffered. But those who persevere in the use of wholesome food will, after a time, find it palatable. Its delicate and delicious flavors will be appreciated, and it will be eaten with greater enjoyment than can be derived from unwholesome dainties. And the stomach, in a healthy condition, neither fevered nor overtaxed, can readily perform its task.

In order to maintain health, a sufficient supply of good, nourishing food is needed. There should not be a great variety at any one meal, for this encourages overeating and causes indigestion.

The meals should be varied. The same dishes, prepared in the same way, should not appear on the table meal after meal and day after day. The meals are eaten with greater relish, and the system is better nourished, when the food is varied.

It is wrong to eat merely to gratify the appetite, but no indifference should be manifested regarding the quality of the food or the manner of its preparation. If the food eaten is not appealing, the body will not be so well nourished. The food should be carefully chosen and prepared with intelligence and skill.

For use in breadmaking, the superfine white flour is not the best. Its use is neither healthful nor economical. Fine-flour bread is lacking in nutritive elements to be found in bread made from the whole wheat. It is a frequent cause of constipation and other unhealthful conditions.

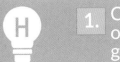 **1.** Choose whole grains over processed, refined grains.

Far too much sugar is ordinarily used in food. Cakes, sweet puddings, pastries, jellies, jams, are active causes of indigestion. Especially harmful are the custards and puddings in which milk, eggs, and sugar are the chief ingredients. The free use of milk and sugar taken together should be avoided.

 2. Careful with the sugar! Especially avoid the combination of sugar and dairy.

If milk is used, it should be thoroughly sterilized; with this precaution, there is less danger of contracting disease from its use. Butter is less harmful when eaten on cold bread than when used in cooking; but, as a rule, it is better to dispense with it altogether. Cheese is still more objectionable; it is wholly unfit for food.

 3. Cut back on the cheese and the butter.

Scanty, poorly-cooked food depraves the blood by weakening the blood-making organs. It deranges the system and brings on disease, with its accompaniment of irritable nerves and bad tempers. The victims of poor cookery are numbered by thousands and tens of thousands. Over many graves might be written: "Died because of poor cooking;" "Died of an abused stomach."

It is a sacred duty for those who cook to learn how to prepare healthful food. Many souls are lost as the result of poor cookery. It takes thought and care to make good bread; but there is more religion in a loaf of good bread than many think. There are few really good cooks.

Cooking is no inferior science, and it is one of the most essential in practical life. To make food appetizing and at the same time simple and nourishing, requires skill; but it can be done. Cooks should know how to prepare simple food in a simple and healthful manner, and so that it will be found more palatable, as well as more wholesome, because of its simplicity.

Regularity in eating is of vital importance. There should be a specified time for each meal. At this time let everyone eat what the system requires and then take nothing more until the next meal. There are many who eat when the system needs no food, at irregular intervals, and between meals, because they have not sufficient strength of will to resist inclination. When traveling, some are constantly nibbling if anything eatable is within their reach. This is very injurious. If travelers would eat regularly of food that is simple and nutritious, they would not feel so great weariness nor suffer so much from sickness.

4. Eat at set times and no snacking!

Another pernicious habit is that of eating just before bedtime. The regular meals may have been taken; but because there is a sense of faintness, more food is eaten. By indulgence this wrong practice becomes a habit and often so firmly fixed that it is thought impossible to sleep without food. As a result of eating late suppers, the digestive process is continued through the sleeping hours. But though the stomach works constantly, its work is not properly accomplished. The sleep is often disturbed with unpleasant dreams, and in the morning the person awakes unrefreshed and with little appetite for breakfast. When we lie down to rest, the stomach should have its work all done, that it, as well as the other organs of the body, may enjoy rest. For persons of sedentary habits, late suppers are particularly harmful. With them the disturbance created is often the beginning of disease that ends in death.

5. Avoid eating close to bed time.

In many cases the faintness that leads to a desire for food is felt because the digestive organs have been too severely taxed during the day. After disposing of one meal, the digestive organs need rest. At least five or six hours should intervene between the meals, and most persons

Eating at regular times with no additional snacks will help your digestive system get a break and will help to improve your overall health.

Some eating patterns that may increase the risk of developing type 2 diabetes in men: [1]

- Skipping breakfast
- Eating frequently
- Snacking

The same study also indicated that snacking and skipping breakfast could contribute to the problem of obesity. [2]

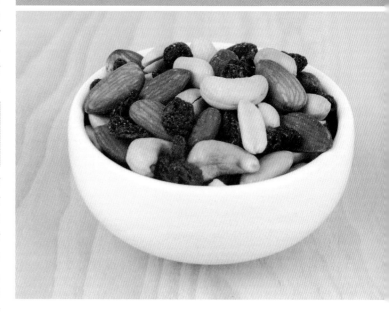

who give the plan a trial will find that two meals a day are better than three.

Food should not be eaten very hot or very cold. If food is cold, the vital force of the stomach is drawn upon in order to warm it before digestion can take place. Cold drinks are injurious for the same reason; while the free use of hot drinks is debilitating. In fact, the more liquid there is taken with the meals, the more difficult it is for the food to digest; for the liquid must be absorbed before digestion can begin. Do not eat largely of salt, avoid the use of pickles and spiced foods, eat an abundance of fruit, and the irritation that calls for so much drink at mealtime will largely disappear.

Food should be eaten slowly and should be thoroughly chewed. This is necessary in order that the saliva may be properly mixed with the food and the digestive fluids be called into action.

6. Chew your food thoroughly.

Another serious evil is eating at improper times, as after violent or excessive exercise, when one is much exhausted or heated. Immediately after eating there is a strong drain upon the nervous energies; and when mind or body is heavily taxed just before or just after eating, digestion is hindered. When one is excited, anxious, or hurried, it is better not to eat until rest or relief is found.

The stomach is closely related to the brain; and when the stomach is diseased, the nerve power is called from the brain to the aid of the weakened digestive organs. When these demands are too frequent, the brain becomes congested. When the brain is constantly taxed, and there is lack of physical exercise, even plain food should be eaten sparingly. At mealtime cast off care and anxious thought; do not feel hurried, but eat slowly and with cheerfulness, with your heart filled with gratitude to God for all His blessings.

7. Make meal time a happy time.

Many who discard flesh meats and other injurious articles think that because their food is simple and wholesome they may indulge appetite without restraint, and they eat to excess, sometimes to gluttony. This is an error. The digestive organs should not be burdened with a quantity or quality of food which it will burden the system to appropriate.

Custom has decreed that the food shall be placed upon the table in courses. Not knowing what is coming next, one may eat a sufficiency of food which perhaps is not the best suited to him. When the last course is brought on, he often ventures to overstep the bounds, and take the tempting dessert, which, however, proves anything but good for him. If all the food intended for a meal is placed on the table at the beginning, one has opportunity to make the best choice.

Sometimes the result of overeating is felt at once. In other cases there is no sensation of pain; but the digestive organs lose their vital force, and the foundation of physical strength is undermined.

The surplus food burdens the system and produces morbid, feverish conditions. It calls an undue amount of blood to the stomach, causing the limbs and extremities to chill quickly. It lays a heavy tax on the digestive organs, and when these organs have accomplished their task, there is a feeling of faintness or weakness. Some who are continually overeating call this all-gone feeling hunger; but it is caused by the over-worked condition of the digestive organs. At times there is numbness of the brain, with disinclination to mental or physical effort.

These unpleasant symptoms are felt because nature has accomplished her work at an unnecessary outlay of vital force and is thoroughly exhausted. The stomach is saying, "Give me rest." But with many the faintness is interpreted as a demand for more food; so instead of giving the stomach rest, another burden is placed upon it. As a consequence the digestive organs are often worn out when they should be capable of doing good work.

Where wrong habits of diet have been indulged, there should be no delay in reform. The stomach may never entirely recover health after long abuse; but a proper course of diet will save further debility, and many will recover more or less fully. It is not easy to prescribe rules that will meet every case; but, with attention to right principles in eating, great reforms may be made, and the cook need not be continually toiling to tempt the appetite.

Restraint in diet is rewarded with mental and moral vigor; it also aids in the control of the passions. Overeating is especially harmful to those who are sluggish in temperament; these should eat sparingly and take plenty of physical exercise. There are men and women of excellent natural ability who do not accomplish half what they might

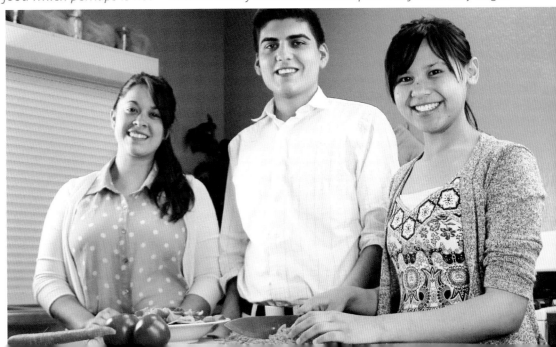

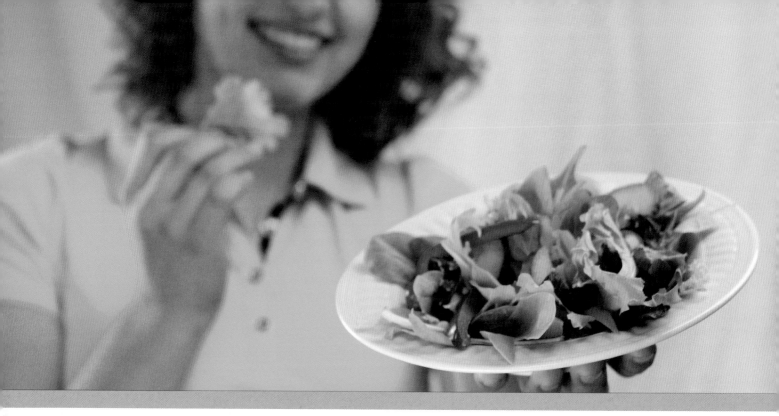

if they would exercise self-control in the denial of appetite.

Many writers and speakers fail here. After eating heartily, they give themselves to sedentary occupations, reading, study, or writing, allowing no time for physical exercise. As a consequence the free flow of thought and words is checked. They cannot write or speak with the force and intensity necessary in order to reach the heart; their efforts are tame and fruitless.

Those upon whom rest important responsibilities, those, above all, who are guardians of spiritual interests, should be men of keen feeling and quick perception. More than others, they need to be temperate in eating. Rich and luxurious food should have no place upon their tables.

Every day men in positions of trust have decisions to make upon which depend results of great importance. Often they have to think rapidly, and this can be done successfully by those only who practice strict temperance. The mind strengthens under the correct treatment of the physical and mental powers. If the strain is not too great, new vigor comes with every such exertion. But often the work of those who have important plans to consider and important decisions to make is affected for evil by the results of improper diet. A disordered stomach produces a disordered, uncertain state of mind. Often it causes irritability, harshness, or injustice. Many a plan that would have been a blessing to the world has been set aside, many unjust, oppressive, even cruel measures have been carried, as the result of diseased conditions due to wrong habits of eating.

Here is a suggestion for all whose work is sedentary or chiefly mental; let those who have sufficient moral courage and self-control try it: At each meal take only two or three kinds of simple food, and eat no more than is required to satisfy hunger. Take active exercise every day, and see if you do not receive benefit.

Strong men who are engaged in active physical labor are not compelled to be as careful as to the quantity or quality of their food as are persons of sedentary habits; but even these would have better health if they would practice self-control in eating and drinking.

Some wish that an exact rule could be prescribed for their diet. They overeat, and then regret it, and so they keep thinking about what they eat and drink. This is not as it should be. One person cannot lay down an exact rule for another. Everyone should exercise reason and self-control, and should act from principle.

Our bodies are Christ's purchased possession, and we are not at liberty to do with them as we please. All who understand the laws of health should realize their obligation to obey these laws which God has established in their being. Obedience to the laws of health is to be made a matter of personal duty. We ourselves must suffer the results of violated law. We must individually answer to God for our habits and practices. Therefore the question with us is not, "What is the world's practice?" but, "How shall I as an individual treat the habitation that God has given me?" ~ The Ministry of Healing, pages 295-310.

HENRY & ANNA
IMPROVED MEAL PLAN

There are many changes that Henry and Anna could make to have a more healthful diet. Here is a sample menu of what a day of healthful eating may look like for them.

Anna's improved weekday of eating may look like this:

Breakfast: An apple, other fruits, whole wheat toast with almond butter and/or oatmeal with fruits and nuts.

Mid-morning break: a tall glass of water with squeezed lemon.

Lunch: A meal from the cafeteria. (Try to opt for the vegetarian option with lots of vegetables. If there are none, go for the option with the most amount of vegetables and least amount of meat, or better yet, pack a lunch!)

Late-afternoon break: Another tall glass of water with squeezed lemon.

Dinner: If too tired to cook, she could try heating up the precooked homemade meals that were made and frozen on Sunday! (See list below for recommended recipes.) If they didn't make any meals ahead of time and must order take-out or eat out, they can choose options that are more healthful with lots of vegetables.

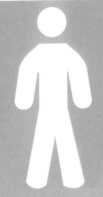

Henry's improved weekday of eating may look like this:

Breakfast: An apple, other fruits, whole wheat toast with almond butter and/or oatmeal with fruits and nuts.

Mid-morning break: A tall glass of water with squeezed lemon.

Lunch: A vegetarian avocado sub sandwich with non-fried chips and no soda.

Late-afternoon break: Another tall glass of water with squeezed lemon.

Dinner: Same as Anna. See above.

With the recipes below, cutting out the meat and dairy may be easier than you think! Many of these recipes can also be made ahead of time and frozen to be eaten at a later time. If it is still absolutely difficult, make small changes at a time such as increasing the amount of vegetables and fruits you eat and cutting back on the amount of meat and dairy.

RECOMMENDED COOKBOOKS - - - - - - - - - - - -

Here is a list of cookbooks for easy, quick, delicious vegetarian meals:

-7 Secrets
-Naturally Gourmet
-Something Better
-The New Life Challenge

-Amazing Health Cookbook
-Kidlicious (kid-friendly recipes that your children can make)
-From Plant to Plate

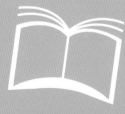

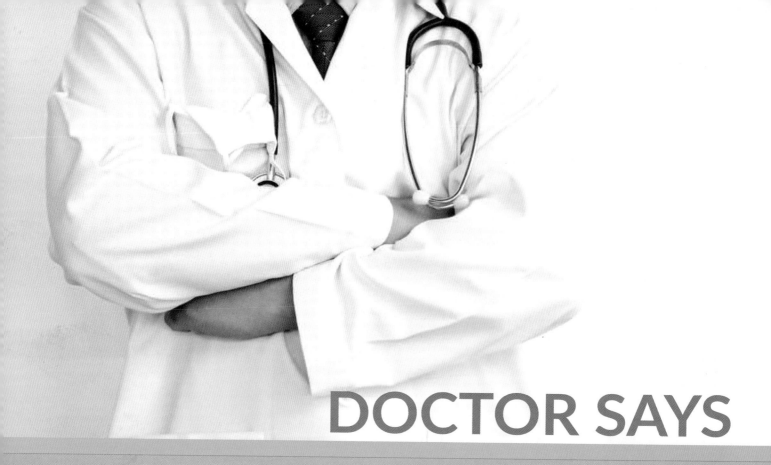

DOCTOR SAYS

As a general rule, if you **DO NOT** have any special health needs or disorders, follow this:

What to eat and drink:

- Fruits, vegetables, beans, grains, nuts, water.

Avoid eating these:

- Meats, poultry, fish, cheese, other animal products, high-sugar, high-fat, high salt, highly processed foods, caffeine, alcohol.

Other Tips:

- Schedule in time to cook. Learn how to cook simple foods.

- Eat a healthful, fulfilling breakfast.

- Eat at specified times and avoid snacking between meals.

- Avoid eating anything 3-4 hours prior to bedtime.

- Eat with other people as much as possible at home.

- Take time to enjoy your food. Chew thoroughly.

- Don't eat while you're angry, stressed, overly excited, etc. Make mealtime a happy time!

- Eat foods close to their natural state as much as possible. (For example: a fresh cluster of grapes is healthier to eat than highly processed, sugary grape jelly.)

- Don't overeat.

TESTIMONIAL
Andrea

My name is Andrea. I am 23 years old. My life was pretty "normal" until I was 13. Around that time, I started to experience weird pains in my hands and feet, but I just dismissed them as growing pains. As the pain grew worse, I visited various doctors and specialists and was diagnosed with rheumatoid arthritis at the young age of 14. The pain eventually became so bad that the rheumatologist recommended a very strong medication, but my parents decided to explore natural ways of healing before giving me that medication.

I am arthritis free! I never dreamed that I would be healed from this painful disease!

One of the first things that my naturopathic doctor recommended was changing my diet. I stopped eating junk foods, avoided sugary foods, and went on a complete plant-based diet. My parents made me healthful juices from lemons and celery in the mornings. They also lovingly cared for my aching joints with hot-and-cold water pads to ease the pain. I also developed a habit of going to bed by 9:30 P.M. and waking up at 6:00 A.M. to help decrease the inflammation and the stiffness by getting enough rest.

Throughout this whole time, so many people prayed for me and helped me. Our family stayed optimistic that I would be able to live a normal life again. There were times when I had to be limited to a wheelchair, and resembled a frail elderly person in a teenager's body. Eventually I started taking the medication that my rheumatologist had suggested and that also helped to alleviate the pain. Throughout this stage of recovery,

not only did change happen externally, but I also started to change on the inside. I began to view my parents as my loving caretakers and my siblings as my dear friends. I also started to make wrongs right with my friends. I developed a deeper relationship with God and began to trust Him and to lovingly rely on Him more and more. These changes within me also paved the road to recovery by developing in me an inner strength of resilience and perseverance.

With these lifestyle changes, supportive family and friends, and an optimistic and trusting attitude, I started to improve. Looking back at the last ten years of my life, I am amazed at how far I have come with the help of God, my family, and friends. Today, as long as I keep following these healthy habits, I am arthritis-free! I never dreamed that I would be healed from this painful disease!

Today, Andrea is studying to become a dietitian with the hope of being able to help others find healing from many diet-related diseases.

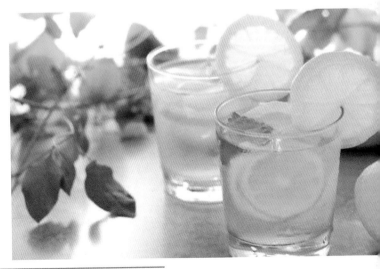

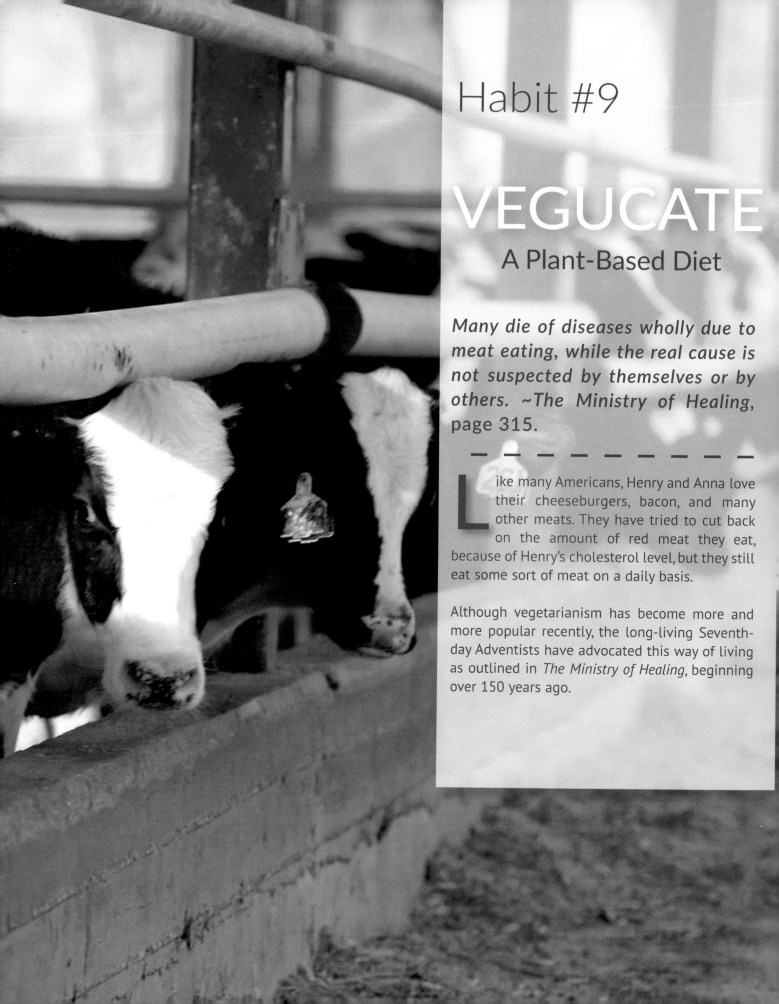

Habit #9

VEGUCATE
A Plant-Based Diet

Many die of diseases wholly due to meat eating, while the real cause is not suspected by themselves or by others. ~The Ministry of Healing, page 315.

— — — — — — — — —

Like many Americans, Henry and Anna love their cheeseburgers, bacon, and many other meats. They have tried to cut back on the amount of red meat they eat, because of Henry's cholesterol level, but they still eat some sort of meat on a daily basis.

Although vegetarianism has become more and more popular recently, the long-living Seventh-day Adventists have advocated this way of living as outlined in *The Ministry of Healing*, beginning over 150 years ago.

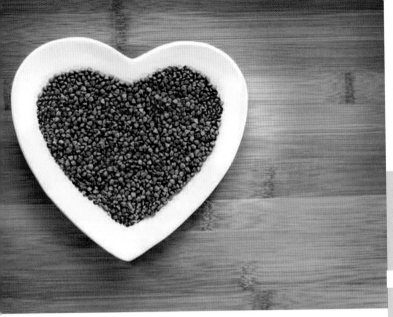

24%

Vegetarians had 24% less risk of dying from coronary heart disease.[1]

20-35%

A balanced vegetarian diet with fiber, soy, and nuts had 20-35% reduced cholesterol level.[2]

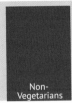

3X

Vegetarians

Non-Vegetarians

Non-vegetarians were 3 times more likely to develop diabetes than vegetarians.[3]

8.5X

A study in Japan showed that women who eat meat daily are 8.5 times more likely to develop breast cancer than those who rarely or never eat meat. [4]

40%

Studies in England and Germany showed that vegetarians were about 40% less likely to develop cancer compared to meat eaters. [5]

The quote below seems to describe a balanced vegetarian or vegan diet. Most, if not all, of the long-living Seventh-day Adventists follow a balanced vegetarian or vegan diet.

As mentioned in the previous chapter:

Grains, fruits, nuts, and vegetables constitute the diet chosen for us by our Creator. These foods, prepared in as simple and natural a manner as possible, are the most healthful and nourishing. They impart a strength, a power of endurance, and a vigor of intellect that are not afforded by a more complex and stimulating diet. ~ The Ministry of Healing, page 296.

3X - - - - - - - - - - - - - ▶

Study done at Harvard University found that people who ate beef, pork, or lamb daily have approximately 3 times the risk of getting colon cancer compared to those who generally avoid these products.[6]

+3X - - - - - - - - - - - - ▶

Those who ate white meat, particularly chicken, have approximately 3 times the risk of getting colon cancer compared to vegetarians.[7]

According to a study published in the *Journal of the American Medical Association*, vegetarian diets are associated with lower risk of [earlier] death. They are also associated with lower risk of many chronic diseases, including hypertension, diabetes, and ischemic heart disease. Such diets also helped to reduce many risk factors of many other diseases, such as stroke, heart disease, and diabetes.[8]

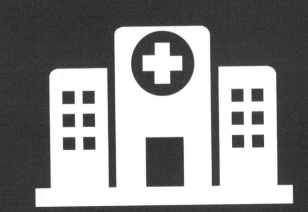

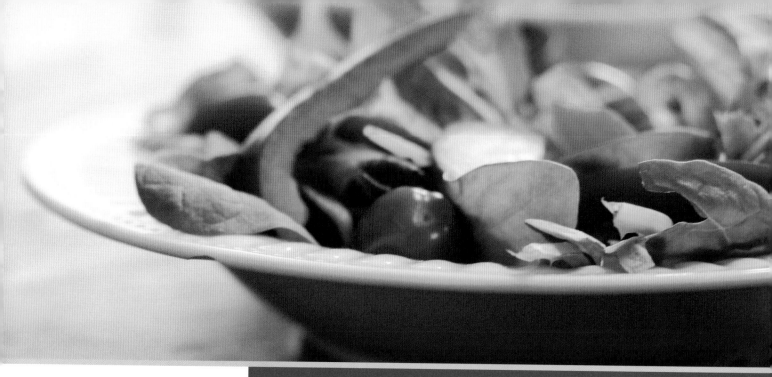

VEGAN DIET

32-44%

Vegans had a 32-44% lower total and LDL cholesterol level than omnivores. [9]

IN CONCLUSION SOMEBODY ON A PLANT-BASED DIET TENDS TO HAVE:[10]

- A healthier body weight
- Lower cholesterol level
- Lower blood pressure
- Lower risk of heart disease
- Lower risk of diabetes
- Lower risk of cancer

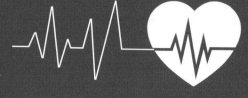

The diet appointed man in the beginning did not include animal food. Not till after the Flood, when every green thing on the earth had been destroyed, did man receive permission to eat flesh.

In choosing man's food in Eden, the Lord showed what was the best diet; in the choice made for Israel He taught the same lesson. He brought the Israelites out of Egypt and undertook their training, that they might be a people for His own possession. Through them He desired to bless and teach the world. He provided them with the food best adapted for this purpose, not flesh, but manna, "the bread of heaven." It was only because of their discontent and their murmuring for the fleshpots of Egypt that animal food was granted them, and this only for a short time. Its use brought disease and death to thousands. Yet the restriction to a nonflesh diet was never heartily accepted. It continued to be the cause of discontent and murmuring, open or secret, and it was not made permanent.

Upon their settlement in Canaan, the Israelites were permitted the use of animal food, but under careful restrictions which tended to lessen the evil results. The use of swine's flesh was prohibited, as also of other animals and of birds and fish whose flesh was pronounced unclean.* Of the meats permitted, the eating of the fat and the blood was strictly forbidden.

Only such animals could be used for food as were in good condition. No creature that was torn, that had died of itself, or from which the blood had not been carefully drained, could be used as food.

By departing from the plan divinely appointed for their diet, the Israelites suffered great loss. They desired a flesh diet, and they reaped its results. They did not reach God's ideal of character or fulfill His purpose. The Lord "gave them their request; but sent leanness into their soul." Psalm 106:15. They valued the earthly above the spiritual, and the sacred pre-eminence which was His purpose for them they did not attain.

Those who eat flesh are but eating grains and vegetables at second hand; for the animal receives from these things the nutrition that produces growth. The life that was in the grains and vegetables passes into the eater. We receive it by eating the flesh of the animal. How much better to get it direct, by eating the food that God provided for our use!

*See Leviticus 11 for a list of the "unclean" and "clean" animals.

Flesh was never the best food; but its use is now doubly objectionable, since disease in animals is so rapidly increasing. Those who use flesh foods little know what they are eating. Often if they could see the animals when living and know the quality of the meat they eat, they would turn from it with loathing. People are continually eating flesh that is filled with tuberculous and cancerous germs. Tuberculosis, cancer, and other fatal diseases are thus communicated.

From Mad Cow Disease to Salmonella to Pink Slime, the safety and cleanliness of the meats being served today are becoming increasingly dangerous and questionable. Be informed and think before you eat that tempting cheeseburger!

Mad Cow Disease: (known as vCJD in humans): This brain-wasting disease became more publicized in the 1990s. It is said to have spread from feeding seemingly healthy cows carcasses of the diseased cows. This disease has been seen in multiple species of animals as well as in humans. The brain starts degenerating into what resembles a porous sponge, the infected person starts having difficulty speaking, stumbling, acting "mad," and eventually dies. There is currently no known cure for this terrifying disease.[11] There is some controversy as to how this disease is transferred, whether through infected meat, milk, gelatin, or other beef products. But many will agree that the best and surest way to prevent this disease is to stay away from beef products.

Salmonella Poisoning: Salmonella bacteria can contaminate foods, especially beef, poultry, milk, and eggs through unsanitary handling. Poisoned symptoms include diarrhea, fever, and abdominal cramps. Many people can recover without treatment, but some may need hospitalization. In some cases, death is the result.[12,13]

Pink Slime: This is a cheap additive in many ground beef products at supermarkets, fast food restaurants, and even school lunches. This is often labeled as 'finely textured beef' or 'boneless lean beef trimmings' but is actually the leftover parts of a cow that normally would not be eaten. These parts tend to be infested with E. coli and other deadly bacteria, so the product is treated with ammonia, and served as hamburgers.[14,15]

These are just three examples of the countless ways that the diseases in the animals and the way we handle the meats could pose a deadly threat to our health.

The tissues of the swine swarm with parasites. Of the swine God said, "It is unclean unto you: ye shall not eat of their flesh, nor touch their dead carcass." Deuteronomy 14:8. This command was given because swine's flesh is unfit for food. Swine are scavengers, and this is the only use they were intended to serve. Never, under any circumstances, was their flesh to be eaten by human beings. It is impossible for the flesh of any living creature to be wholesome when filth is its natural element and when it feeds upon every detestable thing.

According to a report published in January 2013 by *Consumer Reports*, there are some serious concerns about the safety of eating pork.[16] Nearly 70 percent of the pork tested was found to be infected by the bacteria known as Yersinia enterocolitica that can cause fever, diarrhea, and abdominal pain. This bacterium infects about 100,000 Americans a year, especially children. They also found salmonella, staphylococcus aureus, and enterococcus, which can cause similar health problems in humans, including urinary-tract infections. Nearly 90 percent of the pork samples tested had bacteria that were resistant to one or more antibiotics, and 40 percent of the samples had bacteria that were resistant to two to five kinds of antibiotics. This is troubling news because if these bacteria make us sick, the doctors will need to prescribe more powerful antibiotics, contributing to the accelerating growth of drug-resistant "superbugs" that threaten human health.

Although getting infected by the parasite trichinosis used to be the main fear when it came to eating pork, it seems that there are other health concerns to be aware of now. The long-living Seventh-day Adventists have especially avoided eating any type of pork. Maybe there is more wisdom than we realize when God said that it is unclean to eat pigs.

And some of the processes of fattening them [the animals] for market produce disease. Shut away from the light and pure air, breathing the atmosphere of filthy stables, perhaps fattening on decaying food, the entire body soon becomes contaminated with foul matter.

Animals are often transported long distances and subjected to great suffering in reaching a market. Traveling for weary miles over the hot, dusty roads, or crowded into filthy railroad cars, feverish and exhausted, often for many hours deprived of food and water, the poor creatures are driven to their death, that human beings may feast on the carcasses.

In many places fish become so contaminated by the filth on which they feed as to be a cause of disease. This

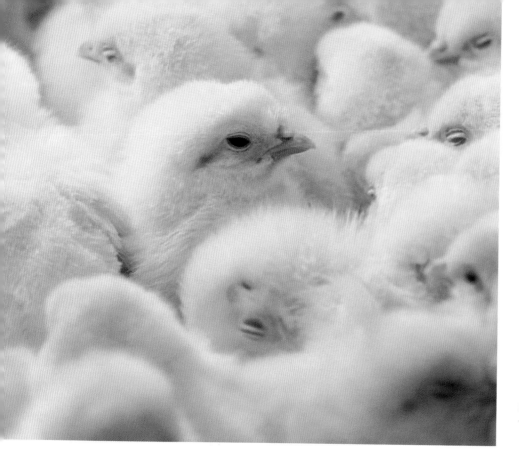

inants that can cause damage to the nervous system, especially in fetuses when the mother consumes them, and various forms of cancer and reproductive problems.[19]

You may be thinking, what about my Omega-3 fatty acids? How will I get that? Isn't fish a healthful option for that? It could be, if there weren't so many negative environmental factors to consider. Omega-3 fatty acids are very important for your brain, heart, and overall health, but it is possible to get these from plant sources that pose a much less health risk from environmental factors.[20] Besides, numerous studies have shown that a well-balanced plant-based diet is much better for your overall health, so you can be healthy even without the fish.

is especially the case where the fish come in contact with the sewage of large cities. The fish that are fed on the contents of the drains may pass into distant waters and may be caught where the water is pure and fresh. Thus when used as food they bring disease and death on those who do not suspect the danger.

In a perfect world without environmental pollution, disease, and unsanitary and crammed fish farms, fish may be an option for dinner. But, considering the circumstances today with water contamination, disease-breeding cramped quarters of industrialized fish farms, and carnivorous fish feed, fish is increasingly becoming a not-so-ideal food for us. Many fish sold at supermarkets and served in restaurants come from industrialized fish farms in which fish are crammed into tight spaces and fed fish feed which usually consists of other dead fish, fish meal, corn, soy, etc., and antibiotics to stave off the diseases which are so easily fostered in these cramped quarters. Even if you consciously choose fish that are wild-caught, it is not unusual for these fish from fish farms to escape into the wild. So, your "wild fish" could very well be a fish from a fish farm or a descendant of a potentially diseased fish from a fish farm.[17,18]

To add to these health risks, there is the problem of mercury, dioxins, PCBs, and other heavy metals and contaminants. Many fish have high levels of these contam-

The effects of a flesh diet may not be immediately realized; but this is no evidence that it is not harmful. Few can be made to believe that it is the meat they have eaten which has poisoned their blood and caused their suffering. Many die of diseases wholly due to meat eating, while the real cause is not suspected by themselves or by others.

The moral evils of a flesh diet are not less marked than are the physical ills. Flesh food is injurious to health, and whatever affects the body has a corresponding effect on the mind and the soul. Think of the cruelty to animals that meat eating involves, and its effect on those who inflict and those who behold it. How it destroys the tenderness with which we should regard these creatures of God!

The intelligence displayed by many animals approaches so closely to human intelligence that it is a mystery. The animals see and hear and love and fear and suffer. They use their organs far more faithfully than many human beings use theirs. They manifest sympathy and tenderness toward their companions in suffering. Many animals show an affection for those who have charge of them, far superior to the affection shown by some of the human race. They form attachments for man which are not broken without great suffering to them.

What man with a human heart, who has ever cared for domestic animals, could look into their eyes, so full of confidence and affection, and willingly give them over to the butcher's knife? How could he devour their flesh as a sweet morsel?

Just search online for "Can animals for meat feel and suffer," "meat cruelty," "factory farming facts" or other similar word variations, and numerous articles and videos will pop up exposing how much animals suffer in order for humans to have their meat. You can also watch the video entitled, "If Slaughterhouses Had Glass Walls, Everyone Would Be Vegetarian."

A large majority of the meat sold in supermarkets and served in restaurants comes from what is called factory farms. The animals are born, caged, and raised indoors in a factory-like setting and killed, cut, packaged, and sold in a systematic manner for maximum financial efficiency. To keep the price of meat low, these are some of the common practices in factory farms: [21,22]

CHICKENS IN FACTORY FARMS [23]

Egg-Laying Hens:

- Up to 10 hens are packed together in one wire cage roughly the size of a file drawer.
- Each bird has less than the area of one 8.5" by 11" sheet of paper to spend its entire lifetime.
- As a result of this close confinement, these hens can go insane and fight each other; to lessen the effects of this problem a portion of the hens' beaks are painfully burned or sliced off with no painkillers.
- A large number of these hens become sick and are either killed or left to die slowly.

Meat Chickens:

- These chickens also live in cramped conditions and are fed excessively and with restricted exercise to grow them as quickly as possible. They grow disproportionately large and cannot support their own weight. Some become crippled, unable to reach for food or water.
- To keep them eating and growing, their sleep is restricted by keeping the lights on for most of the day.
- Chickens can live up to ten years old, but these chickens are usually killed by six weeks old.

Male Chicks:

- The male chicks that are hatched that cannot be raised for meat are shortly killed after their birth by grinding, gassing, crushing, or by suffocation.

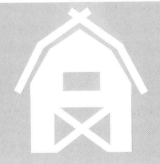

COWS IN FACTORY FARMS[24]

Beef Cows:
- Branded and castrated without painkillers.
- Horns removed without painkillers.
- To increase their weight, fed an unnatural grain diet that is very hard on their bodies, causing illness, pain, and sometimes death.

Veal:
- Are generally taken from their mothers within a day of birth.
- Diets and movements are very restricted to keep their muscles from developing, which makes the meat tender.

Dairy Cows:
- Are given growth hormones, unnatural diets, and are bred selectively to produce about 100 pounds of milk per day—ten times more than their normal amount.
- Many are too sick or injured to stand or walk on their own.
- Experience surgical mutilation with no painkillers.
- Are rampant in mastitis, a painful bacterial infection causing a cow's udder to swell due to unnaturally high milk production.
- To keep the milk flowing, these cows are artificially inseminated once a year. The gestation period lasts nine months, so these cows are pregnant for a majority of their lives.

PIGS AND FISH IN FACTORY FARMS

Pigs:[25]
- Pigs are also kept in extremely cramped and uncomfortable quarters and are artificially inseminated to produce as many piglets as possible for meat.
- Male baby pigs are castrated without painkillers because consumers don't like the smell and taste of uncastrated males.
- Pigs can live up to fifteen years, but most die much earlier due to disease or are killed at just six months.

Many of these animals that are mercilessly killed for food display just as much or sometimes more intelligence, love, and emotions than our pet dog, cat, or even a small child. If we think it is wrong and cruel to treat our pets like this, why is it okay to treat these farm animals in such a way?

It is a mistake to suppose that muscular strength depends on the use of animal food. The needs of the system can be better supplied, and more vigorous health can be enjoyed, without its use. The grains, with fruits, nuts, and vegetables, contain all the nutritive properties necessary to make good blood. These elements are not so well or so fully supplied by a flesh diet. Had the use of flesh been essential to health and strength, animal food would have been included in the diet appointed man in the beginning.

When the use of flesh food is discontinued, there is often a sense of weakness, a lack of vigor. Many urge this as evidence that flesh food is essential; but it is because foods of this class are stimulating, because they fever the blood and excite the nerves, that they are so missed. Some will find it as difficult to leave off flesh eating as it is for the alcoholic to give up his drink; but they will be the better for the change.

When flesh food is discarded, its place should be supplied with a variety of grains, nuts, vegetables, and fruits that will be both nourishing and appetizing. This is especially necessary in the case of those who are weak or who are working continuously. In some countries where poverty abounds, flesh is the cheapest food. Under these circumstances the change will be made with greater difficulty; but it can be effected. We should, however, consider the situation of the people and the

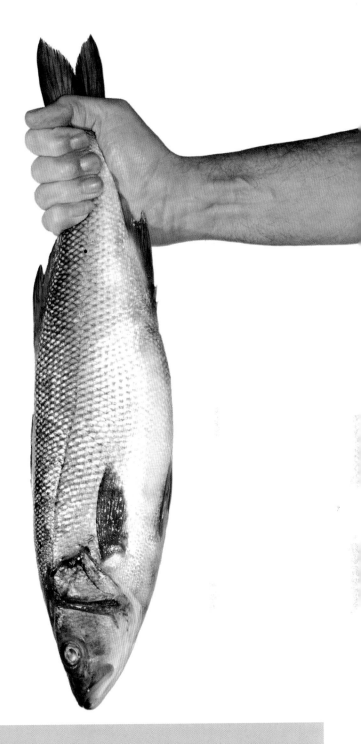

Fish:[26]

- Fish are also kept in extremely tight areas. They are often swimming in waste-filled, murky waters. Disease is rampant, so they are also fed antibiotics.

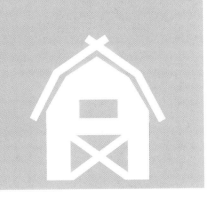

power of lifelong habit, and should be careful not to urge even right ideas unduly. None should be urged to make the change abruptly. The place of meat should be supplied with wholesome foods that are inexpensive.** In this matter very

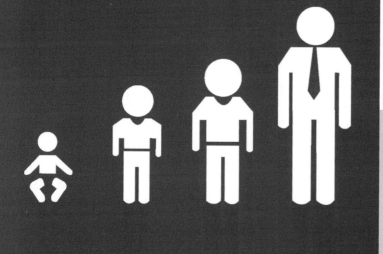

H 1. Go Vegetarian

much depends on the cook. With care and skill, dishes may be prepared that will be both nutritious and appetizing, and will, to a great degree, take the place of flesh food.

In all cases educate the conscience, enlist the will, supply good, wholesome food, and the change will be read-ily made, and the demand for flesh will soon cease.

Is it not time that all should aim to dispense with flesh foods? How can those who are seeking to become pure, refined, and holy, that they may have the companionship of heavenly angels, continue to use as food anything that has so harmful an effect on soul and body? How can they take the life of God's creatures that they may consume the flesh as a luxury? Let them, rather, return to the wholesome and delicious food given to man in the beginning, and themselves practice, and teach their children to practice, mercy toward the creatures that God has made and has placed under our dominion. ~The Ministry of Healing, pages 311-317.

**See the list of vegetarian cookbooks at the end of Habit #8.

Well-planned vegetarian diets are appropriate for all life stages.

"It is the position of the American Dietetic Association that appropriately planned vegetarian diets, including total vegetarian or vegan diets, are healthful, nutritionally adequate, and may provide health benefits in the prevention and treatment of certain diseases. Well-planned vegetarian diets are appropriate for individuals during all stages of the life cycle, including pregnancy, lactation, infancy, childhood, and adolescence, and for athletes." - *Journal of the American Dietetic Association* [27]

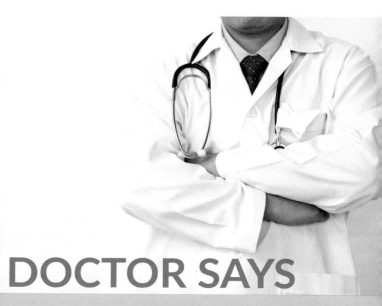

DOCTOR SAYS

Not only is becoming a balanced vegetarian healthier for us, but it is also better for the environment and more humane for the animals.

- If you completely cut out all animal-based foods (meats, chicken, dairy, eggs etc.), make sure you have enough vitamins and minerals such as vitamin B12, calcium, vitamin D, zinc, iron, etc. Many vegetarians/vegans take supplements purchased from the local health food store.

- Make sure to eat a balanced diet. Some helpful books are listed at the end of Habit #8.

- If you are new to vegetarian/vegan cooking and need help or ideas, visit the local Seventh-day Adventist Church or contact them for further assistance.

- Health Ministries Director: katia.reinert@nad.adventist.org
- Website: http://www.nadhealthministries.org/
- Finder: http://www.adventistdirectory.org/

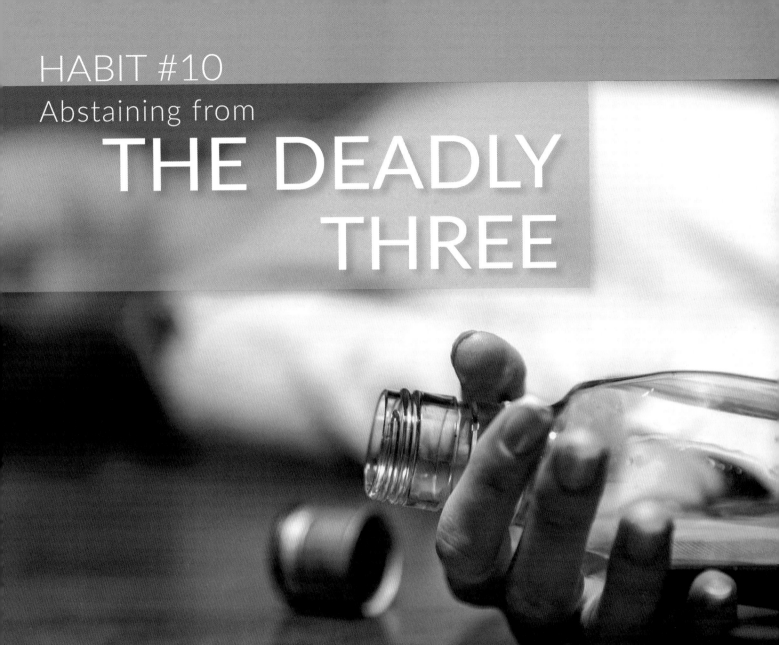

HABIT #10
Abstaining from
THE DEADLY THREE

Henry and Anna both drink about three to four cups of coffee on an average day. They usually don't drink much alcohol on weeknights, but on weekends they like to wind down with some red wine with their dinner. Henry occasionally "treats" himself to some beer and potato chips when his favorite sports team is playing. What they do not realize is by replacing the coffee and alcohol with other ways of getting energized or relaxing, their health could improve greatly. This habit of drinking caffeine and alcohol can be more detrimental than many might think. Read on to learn more.

[Caffeinated] Tea acts as a stimulant, and to a certain extent, produces intoxication. The action of coffee and many other popular drinks is similar. The first effect is exhilarating. The nerves of the stomach are excited; these convey irritation to the brain, and this in turn is stimulated to increase the action of the heart and give short-lived energy to the entire system. Fatigue is forgotten; the strength seems to be increased. The intellect is aroused, the imagination becomes more vivid.

Because of these results, many suppose that their tea or coffee is doing them great good. But this is a mistake. Tea and coffee do not nourish the system. Their effect is produced before there has been time for digestion and assimilation, and what seems to be strength is only nervous excitement. When the influence of the stimulant is gone, the unnatural force abates, and the result is a corresponding degree of languor and debility.

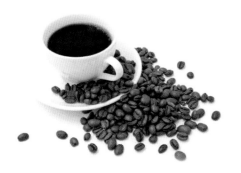

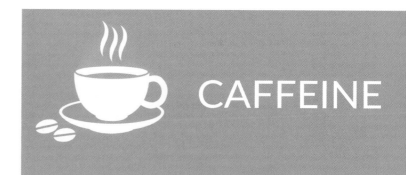

CAFFEINE

The continued use of these nerve irritants is followed by headache, wakefulness, palpitation of the heart, indigestion, trembling, and many other evils; for they wear away the life forces. Tired nerves need rest and quiet instead of stimulation and overwork. Nature needs time to recuperate her exhausted energies. When her forces are goaded on by the use of stimulants, more will be accomplished for a time; but, as the system becomes debilitated by their constant use, it gradually becomes more difficult to rouse the energies to the desired point. The demand for stimulants becomes more difficult to control, until the will is overborne and there seems to be no power to deny the unnatural craving. Stronger and still stronger stimulants are called for, until exhausted nature can no longer respond.

HEALTH EFFECTS OF CAFFEINE

One of the healthy habits of the long-living Seventh-day Adventists is that they stay away from caffeine. Caffeine is a drug that is found in certain plants that can also be man-made and added to foods. It is absorbed and passes quickly into the brain and stimulates, or excites, the brain and the nervous system. It is also a diuretic, a substance that helps to rid your body of fluids, which may lead to dehydration.[1] Many people like to drink caffeinated drinks as a short-term relief for tiredness or drowsiness, but this does not solve the problem of fatigue. In fact, in can lead to or worsen other health problems,[2] such as:

- Anxiety
- Depression
- Sleep problems and insomnia
- Nausea
- Restlessness
- Tremors
- Urinating more often
- Vomiting
- Faster heart rate
- Osteoporosis
- Early death

- Hypertension[3, 4]
- Gout attacks
- Indigestion
- Headaches[5]
- Fertility problems in women[6]
- Diabetes complications[7]
- Worse menopause symptoms[8]
- Tendency to increase the amount of sugary beverages consumed leading to obesity and other health complications[9]

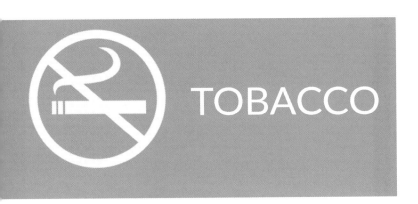

TOBACCO

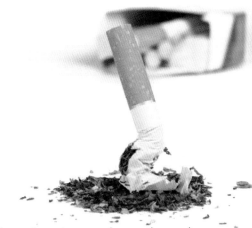

Tobacco is a slow, insidious, but most malignant poison. In whatever form it is used, it tells upon the constitution; it is all the more dangerous because its effects are slow and at first hardly perceptible. It excites and then paralyzes the nerves. It weakens and clouds the brain. Often it affects the nerves in a more powerful manner than does intoxicating drink. It is more subtle, and its effects are difficult to eradicate from the system. Its use excites a thirst for strong drink and in many cases lays the foundation for the liquor habit.

The use of tobacco is inconvenient, expensive, uncleanly, defiling to the user, and offensive to others. It is unpleasant and unhealthful to remain in a room where the atmosphere is laden with the fumes of liquor and tobacco.

Though men persist in using these poisons themselves, what right have they to defile the air that others must breathe?

Among children and youth the use of tobacco is working untold harm. The unhealthful practices of past generations affect the children and youth of today. Mental inability, physical weakness, disordered nerves, and unnatural cravings are transmitted as a legacy from parents to children. And the same practices, continued by the children, are increasing and perpetuating the evil results. In no small degree, this is the reason for the physical, mental, and moral deterioration which is becoming such a cause of alarm.

Secondhand smoke is the combination of smoke from the burning end of a cigarette and the smoke breathed out by smokers. Secondhand smoke contains more than 7,000 chemicals. Hundreds are toxic and about seventy can cause cancer. Since the 1964 Surgeon General's Report, 2.5 million adults who were nonsmokers died because they breathed secondhand smoke.[10]

2.5 Million Died

Secondhand smoke can cause serious health problems in children, such as:[11]

- Bronchitis
- Pneumonia
- Smaller lungs
- Getting sick more often
- Wheezing
- Coughing
- More frequent and severe asthma attacks
- Respiratory infections
- Ear infections
- And numerous other health problems

Some staggering statistics of secondhand smoke:[12]

- Nonsmokers who are exposed to secondhand smoke at home or at work increase their risk of developing heart disease by 25 – 30%.

- Secondhand smoke increases the risk for stroke by 20 – 30%.

- Nonsmokers who are exposed to secondhand smoke at home or at work increase their risk of developing lung cancer by 20 – 30%.

- Smoking during pregnancy results in more than 1,000 infant deaths annually.

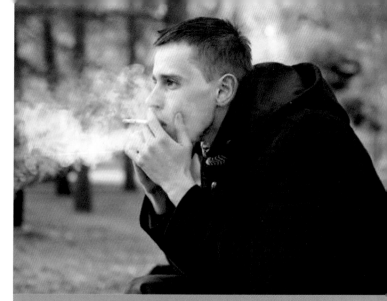

No human being needs tobacco, but multitudes are perishing for want of the means that by its use is worse than wasted. "Know ye not that . . . ye are not your own? For ye are bought with a price: therefore glorify God in your body, and in your spirit, which are God's." 1 Corinthians 6:19, 20.

Smoking is the leading cause of preventable death in the United States.[13]

- About one in five deaths is from cigarette smoking.

- More than 10X as many U.S. citizens have died prematurely from cigarette smoking than have died in all the wars fought by the United States throughout its history.

- Smoking causes about 90% of all lung cancer deaths in men and women. More women die from lung cancer each year than from breast cancer.

- About 80% of all deaths from chronic obstructive pulmonary disease (COPD) are caused by smoking.

Cigarette smoking increases risk for death from all causes in men and women.

Smoking is estimated to increase the risk—[14]

- For coronary heart disease by 2-4X

- For stroke by 2-4X

- Of men developing lung cancer by 25X

- Of women developing lung cancer by 25.7X

- For diabetes by 30-40%

Smoking causes diminished overall health, such as self-reported poor health, increased absenteeism from work, and increased health care utilization and cost.

Smoking causes cancer almost anywhere in your body [15]

- Bladder
- Blood (acute myeloid leukemia)
- Cervix
- Colon and rectum (colorectal)
- Esophagus
- Kidney and ureter
- Larynx
- Liver
- Oropharynx (includes parts of the throat, tongue, soft palate, and the tonsils)
- Pancreas
- Stomach
- Trachea, bronchus, and lung

Smoking and Other Health Risks:[16]

- Fertility problems and increased risk for birth defects and miscarriages
- Stillbirth
- Low birth weight
- Pregnancy complications
- Weaker bones
- Poorer teeth and gum health
- Increased risk of cataracts
- Higher risk of developing rheumatoid arthritis
- Inflammation
- Poorer immune function
- Diabetes complications

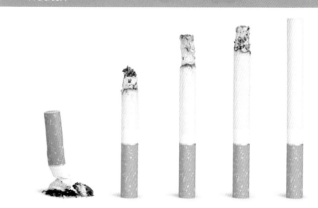

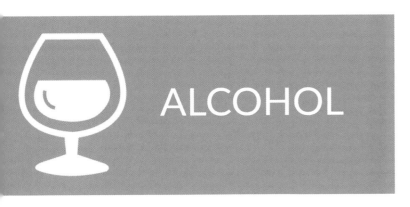

ALCOHOL

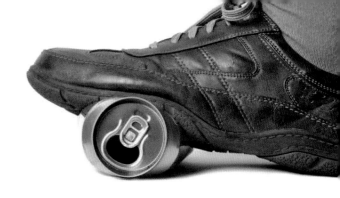

"Wine is a mocker, strong drink is raging:
And whosoever is deceived thereby is not wise."
"Who hath woe? who hath sorrow? who hath conten-
tions?
who hath babbling? who hath wounds
without cause?
Who hath redness of eyes?
They that tarry long at the wine;
They that go to seek mixed wine.
Look not thou upon the wine when it is red,
When it giveth his color in the cup,
When it moveth itself aright.
At the last it biteth like a serpent,
And stingeth like an adder."

— **Proverbs 20:1; 23:29-32.**

Never was traced by human hand a more vivid pic-
ture of the debasement and the slavery of the victim of intox-
icating drink. Enthralled, degraded, even when awakened to a
sense of his misery, he has no power to break from the snare;
he "will seek it yet again." Proverbs 23:35.

And who can picture the wretchedness, the agony,
the despair, that are hidden in the drunkard's home? Think
of the wife, often delicately reared, sensitive, cultured, and
refined, linked to one whom drink transforms into a sot or
a demon. Think of the children, robbed of home comforts,
education, and training, living in terror of him who should
be their pride and protection, thrust into the world, bearing
the brand of shame, often with the hereditary curse of the
drunkard's thirst.

To get a better understanding of how devastating alcoholism is in our country, here are a few figures from the Centers for Disease Control and Prevention (CDC):[17,18]

88,000 deaths are annually attributed to excessive alcohol use.

Excessive alcohol use is responsible for 2.5 million years of potential life lost (YPLL) annually, or an average of about 30 years of potential life lost for each death.

Excessive alcohol consumption cost the U.S. economy about $223.5 billion in 2006.

Alcoholism is the 3rd leading lifestyle-related cause of death in the nation.

Think of the frightful accidents that are every day
occurring through the influence of drink.... To what extent
can one indulge the liquor habit and be safely trusted with
the lives of human beings? He can be trusted only as he
totally abstains.

The Bible nowhere sanctions the use of intoxicating
wine. The wine that Christ made from water at the marriage
feast of Cana was the pure juice of the grape. This is the
"new wine ... found in the cluster," of which the Scripture
says, "Destroy it not; for a blessing is in it." Isaiah 65:8.

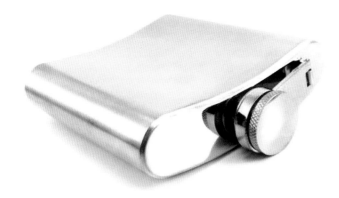

It was Christ who, in the Old Testament, gave the warning to Israel, "Wine is a mocker, strong drink is raging: and whosoever is deceived thereby is not wise." Proverbs 20:1. He Himself provided no such beverage. Satan tempts men to indulgence that will becloud reason and benumb the spiritual perceptions, but Christ teaches us to bring the lower nature into subjection. He never places before men that which would be a temptation. His whole life was an example of self-denial. It was to break the power of appetite that in the forty days' fast in the wilderness He suffered in our behalf the severest test that humanity could endure. It was Christ who directed that John the Baptist should drink neither wine nor strong drink. It was He who enjoined similar abstinence upon the wife of Manoah. Christ did not contradict His own teaching. The unfermented wine that He provided for the wedding guests was a wholesome and refreshing drink. This is the wine that was used by our Savior and His disciples in the first Communion. It is the wine that should always be used on the Communion table as a symbol of the Savior's blood. The sacramental service is designed to be soul-refreshing and life-giving. There is to be connected with it nothing that could minister to evil.

In the light of what the Scriptures, nature, and reason teach concerning the use of intoxicants, how can Christians engage in beer making, or in the manufacture of wine or cider for the market? If they love their neighbor as themselves, how can they help to place in his way that which will be a snare to him?

Often intemperance begins in the home. By the use of rich, unhealthful food the digestive organs are weakened, and a desire is created for food that is still more stimulating. Thus the appetite is educated to crave continually something stronger. The demand for stimulants becomes more frequent and more difficult to resist. The system becomes more or less filled with poison, and the more debilitated it becomes, the greater is the desire for these things. One step in the wrong direction prepares the way for another. Many who would not be guilty of placing on their table wine or liquor of any kind will load their table with food which creates such a thirst for strong drink that to resist the temptation is almost impossible. Wrong habits of eating and drinking destroy the health and prepare the way for drunkenness.

There is work for mothers in helping their children to form correct habits and pure tastes. Educate the appetite; teach the children to abhor stimulants. Bring your children up to have moral stamina to resist the evil that surrounds them. Teach them that they are not to be swayed by others, that they are not to yield to strong influences, but to influence others for good.

It must be kept before the people that the right

balance of the mental and moral powers depends in a great degree on the right condition of the physical system. All narcotics and unnatural stimulants that enfeeble and degrade the physical nature tend to lower the tone of the intellect and morals. Intemperance lies at the foundation of the moral depravity of the world. By the indulgence of perverted appetite, man loses his power to resist temptation.

In relation to tea, coffee, tobacco, and alcoholic drinks, the only safe course is to touch not, taste not, handle not. The tendency of tea, coffee, and similar drinks is in the same direction as that of alcoholic liquor and tobacco, and in some cases the habit is as difficult to break as it is for the drunkard to give up intoxicants. Those who attempt to leave off these stimulants will for a time feel a loss and will suffer without them. But by persistence they will overcome the craving and cease to feel the lack. Nature may require a little time to recover from the abuse she has suffered; but give her a chance, and she will again rally and perform her work nobly and well. ~ The Ministry of Healing, pages 325-335.

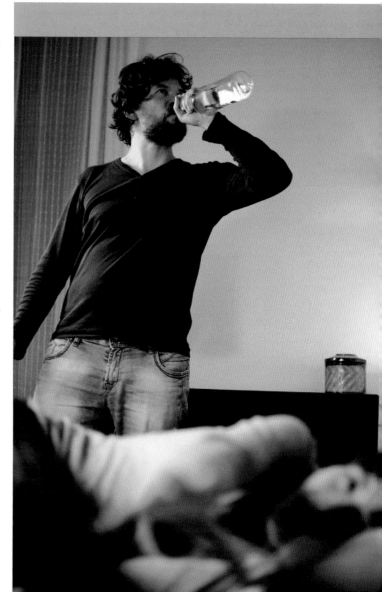

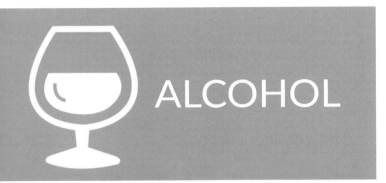

ALCOHOL

"Alcohol abuse and alcoholism can affect all aspects of your life. Long-term alcohol use can cause serious health complications affecting virtually every organ in your body, including your brain. It can also damage your emotional stability, finances, career, and impact your family, friends and the people you work with."[19] —National Council on Alcoholism and Drug Dependence

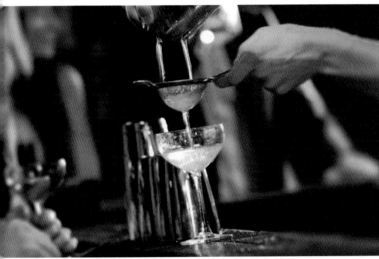

Diseases, Disorders, and Risks associated with Alcohol: [20, 21, 22]

- High Blood Pressure
- Heart Disease
- Stroke
- Liver Disease
- Pancreas Diseases
- Infectious Diseases
- Cancers
  - Breast
  - Mouth
  - Throat
  - Esophagus
  - Liver
  - Colon
- Birth Defects and numerous problems for the unborn baby when the pregnant mother drinks

- Digestive Problems
- Epilepsy
- Learning and Memory Problems
- Poor School Performance
- Dementia
- Mental Health Disorders
  - Depression
  - Anxiety
- Social Problems
  - Lost productivity
  - Family problems
  - Unemployment
  - Violence
- Injuries

H
1. Go caffeine-free.
2. Don't smoke. Stay away from second-hand smoke.
3. Don't drink alcohol.

Beware of being misled by different ideas and misconceptions that seem to imply that toxins such as caffeine, tobacco, and alcohol could be beneficial to your health.

Caffeine is a toxin. Tobacco is a toxin. Alcohol is a toxin. If you are unable to stop or cut back on the usage of caffeine, tobacco, or alcohol, get some professional help.

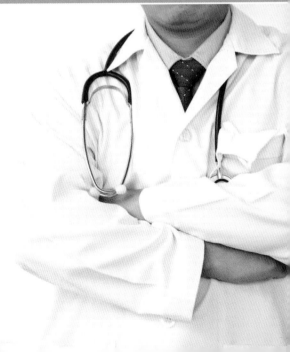

DOCTOR SAYS

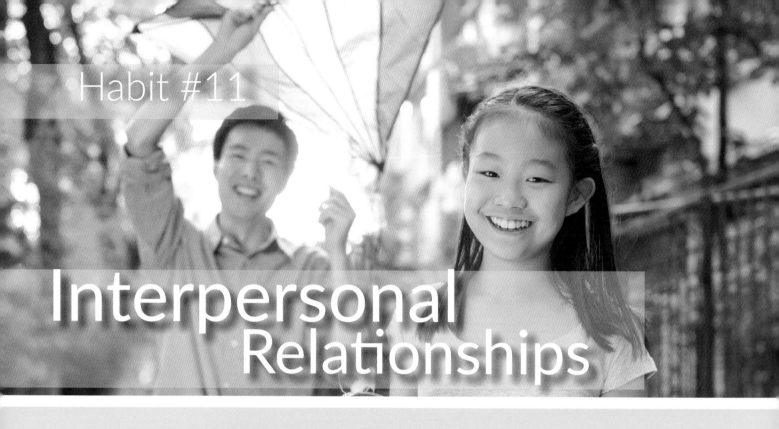

Habit #11

Interpersonal Relationships

When wrongs have been righted, we may present the needs of the sick to the Lord in calm faith, as His Spirit may indicate. He knows each individual by name, and cares for each as if there were not another upon the earth for whom He gave His beloved Son. ~ The Ministry of Healing, page 229.

Anna suffers from mild depression. She usually doesn't sleep well and rarely feels refreshed in the morning. She has tried switching to a more comfortable mattress, but her sleep problems have only worsened throughout the past few years. She is constantly low on energy and has a difficult time staying active. And strangely, she seems to crave many junk foods, especially when she is in her low, depressive state.

She has experienced these symptoms on and off for the past couple decades, especially after tense situations with her coworkers. But it was about five years ago that these symptoms began to intensify dramatically. About five and half years ago she had had a bitter fight with her eldest child and only daughter. Since then, they have maintained a cold, distant relationship. With the passing of years the rift between them has only grown wider, and Anna's depressive symptoms and her health have only worsened.

You may have already guessed it. What Anna should do is resolve the issue in her family. She should make things right with her daughter and try to develop a positive relationship with her.

Every association of life calls for the exercise of self-control, restraint, and sympathy. We differ so widely in disposition, habits, education, that our ways of looking at things vary. We judge differently. Our understanding of truth, our ideas in regard to the conduct of life, are not in all respects the same. There are no two whose experience is alike in every particular. The trials of one are not the trials of another. The duties that one finds light are to another most difficult and perplexing.

Human nature is so frail, so ignorant, and so liable to misunderstandings, that each should be careful in the estimate he places upon another. We little know the bearing of our acts upon the experience of others. What we do or say may seem to us of little significance, when, could our eyes be opened, we should see that upon it depended the most important results for good or for evil.

The Effects of Marital Stress

Here are some studies that show how interconnected our health is with our interpersonal relationships:

Women who reported moderate to severe marital strain were 2.9 times more likely to need heart surgery, suffer heart attacks, or die of heart disease than women without marital stress.[1]

2.9x Worse

Studies have shown that the negative effects of marital stress for women are just as detrimental to health as smoking and physical inactivity.[2]

Worse than Smoking

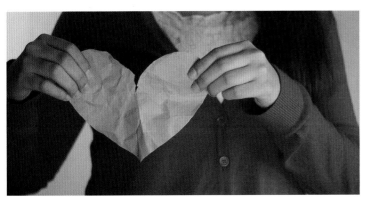

Marital Strain

Those with more marital concerns reported greater stress throughout the day, had higher blood pressure in the middle of the work day and higher morning cortisol levels. Over time, these factors can combine to increase the risk of obesity, diabetes, depression, heart attack, and stroke.[3] Marital conflict has also been linked to weakening of the immune system.[4]

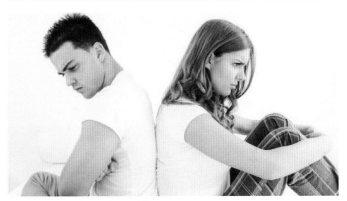

Unhealthy Relationships

Women who experienced more conflicts and disagreements in their relationships also had a higher risk of high blood pressure, abdominal obesity, high blood sugar, high triglycerides and low levels of the "good" HDL cholesterol.[5] The study also found that females were more affected than the males.

We cannot afford to let our spirits chafe over any real or supposed wrong done to ourselves. Self is the enemy we most need to fear. No form of evil has a more harmful effect upon the character than has human passion not under the control of the Holy Spirit. No other victory we can gain will be so precious as the victory gained over self.

We should not allow our feelings to be easily wounded. We are to live, not to guard our feelings or our reputation, but to save souls. As we become interested in the salvation of others, we cease to mind the little differences that so often arise in our association with one another. Whatever they may think of us or do to us, it need not disturb our oneness with Christ, the fellowship of the Spirit. "What glory is it, if, when ye be buffeted for your faults, ye

shall take it patiently? but if, when ye do well, and suffer for it, ye take it patiently, this is acceptable with God." 1 Peter 2:20.

Do not retaliate. So far as you can do so, remove all cause for misunderstanding. Avoid the appearance of evil. Do all that lies in your power, without the sacrifice of principle, to conciliate others. "If thou bring thy gift to the altar, and there rememberest that thy brother hath aught against thee; leave there thy gift before the altar, and go thy way; first be reconciled to thy brother, and then come and offer thy gift." Matthew 5:23, 24.

If impatient words are spoken to you, never reply in the same spirit. Remember that "a soft answer turneth away wrath." Proverbs 15:1. And there is wonderful power in silence. Words spoken in reply to one who is angry some-

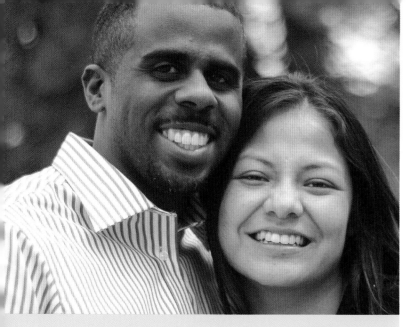

the books, and heaven will take care of them. While we are counting up the disagreeable things, many things that are pleasant to reflect upon are passing from memory, such as the merciful kindness of God surrounding us every moment and the love over which angels marvel, that God gave His Son to die for us. If as workers for Christ you feel that you have had greater cares and trials than have fallen to the lot of others, remember that for you there is a peace unknown to those who shun these burdens. There is comfort and joy in the service of Christ. Let the world see that life with Him is no failure.

If you do not feel lighthearted and joyous, do not talk of your feelings. Cast no shadow upon the lives of others. A cold, sunless religion never draws souls to Christ. It drives them away from Him into the nets that Satan has spread for the feet of the straying. Instead of thinking of your discouragements, think of the power you can claim in Christ's name. Let your imagination take hold upon things unseen. Let your thoughts be directed to the evidences of the great love of God for you. Faith can endure trial, resist temptation, bear up under disappointment. Jesus lives as our advocate. All is ours that His mediation secures.

"Be kindly affectioned one to another with brotherly love; in honor preferring one another." "Not rendering evil for evil, or railing for railing: but contrariwise blessing; knowing that ye are thereunto called, that ye should inherit a blessing." Romans 12:10; 1 Peter 3:9.

The Lord Jesus demands our acknowledgment of the rights of every man. Men's social rights, and their rights as Christians, are to be taken into consideration. All are to be treated with refinement and delicacy, as the sons and daughters of God.

Christianity will make a man a gentleman. Christ was courteous, even to His persecutors; and His true followers will manifest the same spirit. Look at Paul when brought before rulers. His speech before Agrippa is an illustration of true courtesy as well as persuasive eloquence. The gospel does not encourage the formal politeness current with the world, but the courtesy that springs from real kindness of heart.

times serve only to exasperate. But anger met with silence, in a tender, patient spirit, quickly dies away.

Under a storm of stinging, faultfinding words, keep the mind stayed upon the word of God. Let mind and heart be stored with God's promises. If you are ill-treated or wrongfully accused, instead of returning an angry answer, repeat to yourself the precious promises [shown below].

So long as we are in the world, we shall meet with adverse influences. There will be provocations to test the temper; and it is by meeting these in a right spirit that the Christian graces are developed. If Christ dwells in us, we shall be patient, kind, and restrained, cheerful amid frets and irritations. Day by day and year by year we shall conquer self, and grow into a noble heroism. This is our allotted task; but it cannot be accomplished without help from Jesus, resolute decision, unwavering purpose, continual watchfulness, and unceasing prayer. Each one has a personal battle to fight. Not even God can make our characters noble or our lives useful, unless we become co-workers with Him. Those who decline the struggle lose the strength and joy of victory.

We need not keep our own record of trials and difficulties, griefs, and sorrows. All these things are written in

Promises for Everyday Living

"Be not overcome of evil, but overcome evil with good" Romans 12:21.

"Commit thy way unto the Lord; trust also in Him; and He shall bring it to pass. And He shall bring forth thy righteousness as the light, and thy judgment as the noonday" Psalm 37:5, 6.

"There is nothing covered, that shall not be revealed; neither hid, that shall not be known" Luke 12:2.

"Thou hast caused men to ride over our heads; we went through fire and through water: but Thou broughtest us out into a wealthy place" Psalm 66:12.

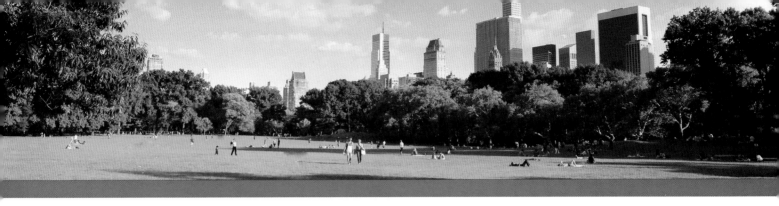

Health is affected not only by marital problems, but by other social relationships as well. According to a study released by the National Institutes of Health, both the quantity and quality of social relationships affect mental health, health behavior, physical health, and mortality risk.[6]

Risk of death among men and women with the fewest social ties was more than twice as high as the risk for adults with the most social ties.[7]

>2X the Risk

Adults with heart disease who were also socially isolated had a 2.4 times greater risk of cardiac death than their more socially connected peers who also had heart disease.[8]

2.4X the Risk

Conditions linked with low quantity or quality of social ties:[9]
- Heart disease
- Atherosclerosis
- High blood pressure
- Cancer & delayed cancer recovery
- Impaired immune function
- Slower wound healing

Loneliness and isolation can increase the likelihood of disease and premature death from all causes by 200% to 500% or more![10]

200-500%

The most careful cultivation of the outward proprieties of life is not sufficient to shut out all fretfulness, harsh judgment, and unbecoming speech. True refinement will never be revealed so long as self is considered as the supreme object. Love must dwell in the heart. Genuine Christians draw their motives of action from their deep heart love for their Master. Up through the roots of their affection for Christ springs an unselfish interest in others. Love imparts to its possessors grace, propriety, and comeliness of deportment. It illuminates the countenance and subdues the voice; it refines and elevates the whole being.

Life is chiefly made up, not of great sacrifices and wonderful achievements, but of little things. It is most often through the little things, which seem so unworthy of notice that great good or evil is brought into our lives. It is through our failure to endure the tests that come to us in little things, that the habits are molded, the character misshaped; and when the greater tests come, they find us

unready. Only by acting upon principle in the tests of daily life can we acquire power to stand firm and faithful in the most dangerous and most difficult positions.

We are never alone. Whether we choose Him or not, we have a companion. Remember that wherever you are, whatever you do, God is there. Nothing that is said or done or thought can escape His attention. To your every word or deed you have a witness—the holy, sin-hating God. Before you speak or act, always think of this. As a Christian, you are a member of the royal family, a child of the heavenly King. Say no word, do no act, that shall bring dishonor upon "that worthy name by the which ye are called." James 2:7.

Study carefully the divine-human character, and constantly inquire, "What would Jesus do were He in my place?" This should be the measurement of our duty. Do not place yourselves needlessly in the society of those who by their influence would weaken your purpose to do right, or bring a stain upon your conscience. Do nothing among strangers, in the street, in travel, in the home, that would have the least appearance of evil. Do something every day to improve, beautify, and ennoble the life that Christ has purchased with His own blood.

Always act from principle, never from impulse. Temper the natural impulsiveness of your nature with meekness and gentleness. Indulge in no lightness or foolishness. Let no low witticism escape your lips. Even the thoughts are not to be allowed to run riot. They must be restrained, brought into captivity to the obedience of Christ. Let them be placed upon holy things. Then, through the grace of Christ, they will be pure and true.

We need a constant sense of the ennobling power of pure thoughts. The only security for any soul is right thinking. As a man "thinketh in his heart, so is he." Proverbs 23:7. The power of self-restraint strengthens by exercise. That which at first seems difficult, by constant repetition grows easy, until right thoughts and actions become habitual. If we will we may turn away from all that is cheap and inferior, and rise to a high standard; we may be respected by men and beloved of God.

Cultivate the habit of speaking well of others. Dwell upon the good qualities of those with whom you associate, and see as little as possible of their errors and failings. When tempted to complain of what someone has said or done, praise something in that person's life or character. Cultivate thankfulness. Praise God for His wonderful love in giving Christ to die for us. It never pays to think of our grievances. God calls upon us to think of His mercy and His matchless love, that we may be inspired with praise.

Earnest workers have no time for dwelling upon the faults of others. We cannot afford to live on the husks of others' faults or failings. Evilspeaking is a twofold curse, falling more heavily upon the speaker than upon the hearer. He who scatters the seeds of dissension and strife reaps in his own soul the deadly fruits. The very act of looking for evil in others develops evil in those who look. By dwelling upon the faults of others, we are changed into the same image. But by beholding Jesus, talking of His love and perfection of character, we become changed into His image. By contemplating the lofty ideal He has placed before us, we shall be uplifted into a pure and holy atmosphere, even the presence of God. When we abide here, there goes forth from us a light that illuminates all who are connected with us.

Instead of criticizing and condemning others, say, "I must work out my own salvation. If I cooperate with Him who desires to save my soul, I must watch myself diligently. I must put away every evil from my life. I must overcome every fault. I must become a new creature in Christ. Then, instead of weakening those who are striving against evil, I can strengthen them by encouraging words." We are too indifferent in regard to one another. Too often we forget that our fellow laborers are in need of strength and cheer. Take care to assure them of your interest and sympathy. Help them by your prayers, and let them know that you do it.

Remember that you cannot read hearts. You do not know the motives which prompted the actions that to you look wrong. There are many who have not received a right education; their characters are warped, they are hard and gnarled, and seem to be crooked in every way. But the grace of Christ can transform them. Never cast them aside, never drive them to discouragement or despair by saying, "You have disappointed me, and I will not try to help you." A few words spoken hastily under provocation—just what we think they deserve—may cut the cords of influence that

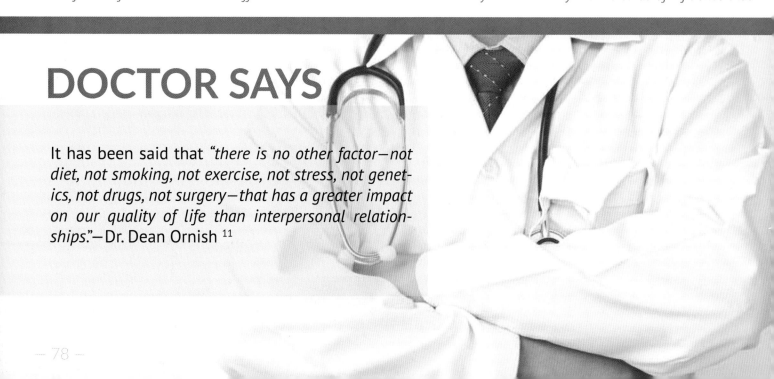

DOCTOR SAYS

It has been said that "there is no other factor—not diet, not smoking, not exercise, not stress, not genetics, not drugs, not surgery—that has a greater impact on our quality of life than interpersonal relationships."—Dr. Dean Ornish [11]

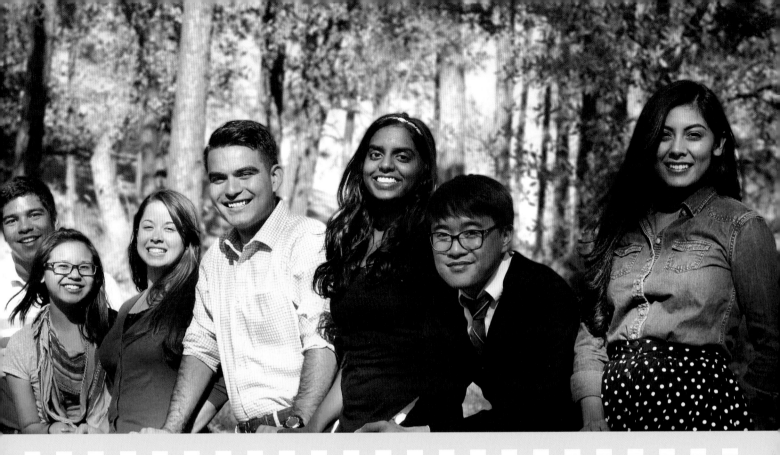

should have bound their hearts to ours.

The consistent life, the patient forbearance, the spirit unruffled under provocation, is always the most conclusive argument and the most solemn appeal. If you have had opportunities and advantages that have not fallen to the lot of others, consider this, and be ever a wise, careful, gentle teacher.

In order to have the wax take a clear, strong impression of the seal, you do not dash the seal upon it in a hasty, violent way; you carefully place the seal on the soft wax and quietly, steadily press it down until it has hardened in the mold. In like manner deal with human souls. The consistency of Christian influence is the secret of its power, and this depends on the steadfastness of your manifestation of the character of Christ. Help those who have erred, by telling them of your experiences. Show how, when you made grave mistakes, patience, kindness, and helpfulness on the part of your fellow workers gave you courage and hope.

Until the judgment you will never know the influence of a kind, considerate course toward the inconsistent, the unreasonable, the unworthy. When we meet with ingratitude and betrayal of sacred trusts, we are roused to show our contempt or indignation. This the guilty expect; they are prepared for it. But kind self-restraint takes them by surprise and often awakens their better impulses and arouses a longing for a nobler life.

"Brethren, if a man be overtaken in a fault, ye which are spiritual, restore such an one in the spirit of meekness; considering thyself, lest thou also be tempted. Bear ye one another's burdens, and so fulfill the law of Christ." Galatians 6:1, 2.

All who profess to be children of God should bear in mind that as missionaries they will be brought into contact with all classes of minds. There are the refined and the coarse, the humble and the proud, the religious and the skeptical, the educated and the ignorant, the rich and the poor. These varied minds cannot be treated alike; yet all need kindness and sympathy. By mutual contact our minds should receive polish and refinement. We are dependent upon one another, closely bound together by the ties of human brotherhood.

It is through the social relations that Christianity comes in contact with the world. Social power, sanctified by the Spirit of Christ, must be improved in bringing people to the Saviour. Christ is not to be hid away in the heart as a coveted treasure, sacred and sweet, to be enjoyed solely by the possessor. We are to have Christ in us as a well of water, springing up into everlasting life, refreshing all who come in contact with us. ~ The Ministry of Healing, pages 483-496.

1. Seek first to understand rather than be understood.

Sadly, some strained relationships are solely due to misunderstandings. Think of a current or past strained relationship. Have you considered what the other person may have felt or thought? Did the other person understand what you were trying to communicate? Have you ever considered that you may have misunderstood what the other person was trying to communicate? In most interpersonal relationships, it helps to think the best of others. In the case of abusive relationships, things will need to be dealt with differently. But, in other situations and relationships, when safe to do so, give others the benefit of the doubt. It could just be a simple misunderstanding.

 2. Be forgiving.

Forgiveness is an interesting thing. Although it is something that can seem so hard to do, especially when you have been very deeply hurt, it is something that can benefit not just the one receiving forgiveness, but especially the one forgiving another. In order to understand what forgiveness is, let's look at what forgiveness is NOT.

What Forgiveness is NOT: [12]
Forgiveness of others does not mean you have to trust them, doesn't mean you're excusing them for what they did, nor does it mean that you are approving their behavior or forgetting what they did. It doesn't necessarily even mean reconciliation.

So, what is Forgiveness?
It has been said that forgiveness is simply surrendering your right to do, wish, or think evil upon the other person.[13] You can choose to forgive. As difficult as it may seem in some situations, you can choose to surrender your "right" to wish hurt or think evil upon the other person.

Many people have described the act of forgiveness as very relieving because it liberates them from their bitterness toward another person. Hanging on to a grudge or bitterness is like drinking poison and expecting the other person to die.[14] Have you let go of any bitterness? Have you forgiven the people in your life that you need to forgive?

 3. Spend time with your loved ones.

Make time for the people that matter the most to you. Write them into your schedule and make it a priority.

 4. Give your loved ones your full attention.

Take a mini "vacation" from technology. Make a rule to put the phone, tablet, and/or laptop away when spending time with your loved ones. Enjoy the simple pleasure of just eating with and/or chatting with the people you care about.

Thoughts: The Power of the Mind

The relation that exists between the mind and the body is very intimate. When one is affected, the other sympathizes. ~The Ministry of Healing, page 241.

Earlier we mentioned how Anna struggles with mild depression. She has battled negative thoughts and depression for decades now, but the symptoms took a turn for the worse about five years ago after a bitter incident with her only daughter. Since then she has experienced more than just negative and debilitating thoughts. She started experiencing other symptoms mentioned in the following chart, such as sleeping problems and pain in her back and shoulder area.

There may very well be other physical disorders that are causing these problems, but it would help Anna to understand how interconnected our mental and emotional well-being is with our physical health. Read on to learn more.

The relation that exists between the mind and the body is very intimate. When one is affected, the other sympathizes. The condition of the mind affects the health to a far greater degree than many realize. Many of the diseases from which people suffer are the result of mental depression. Grief, anxiety, discontent, remorse, guilt, distrust, all tend to break down the life forces and to invite decay and death. ~ The Ministry of Healing, page 241.

Diseases and Health Behaviors associated with Depression:[1, 2]

- Chronic Pain States
- Fibromyalgia
- Chronic Fatigue
- Irritable Bowel Syndrome
- Smoking
- Alcohol Consumption
- Physical Inactivity/ Obesity
- Sleep Disturbance

Disease is sometimes produced, and is often greatly aggravated, by the imagination. Many carry lifelong illnesses who might be well if they only thought so. Many imagine that every slight exposure will cause illness, and the evil effect is produced because it is expected. Many die from disease the cause of which is wholly imaginary. ~ The Ministry of Healing, page 241.

Therefore ...

Courage, hope, faith, sympathy, love, promote health and prolong life. A contented mind, a cheerful spirit, is health to the body and strength to the soul. "A merry heart doeth good like a medicine." Proverbs 17:22. ~ The Ministry of Healing, page 241.

Nothing tends more to promote health of body and of soul than does a spirit of gratitude and praise... . It is a law of nature that our thoughts and feelings are encouraged and strengthened as we give them utterance. While words express thoughts, it is also true that thoughts follow words. ~ The Ministry of Healing, page 251.

And remember this ...

In the treatment of the sick the effect of mental influence should not be overlooked. Rightly used, this influence affords one of the most effective agencies for combating disease. ...

Great wisdom is needed in dealing with diseases caused through the mind. A sore, sick heart, a discouraged mind, needs mild treatment. Many times some living home trouble is, like a canker, eating to the very soul and weakening the life force. And sometimes it is the case that remorse for sin undermines the constitution and unbalances the mind. It is through tender sympathy that this class of sick people can be benefited. The physician should first gain their confidence and then point them to the Great Healer. If their faith can be directed to the True Physician, and they can have confidence that He has undertaken their

Health benefits that positive thinking may provide:[3]

- Increased life span
- Lower rates of depression
- Greater resistance to the common cold
- Better psychological and physical well-being
- Reduced risk of death from cardiovascular disease
- Better coping skills during hardships and times of stress

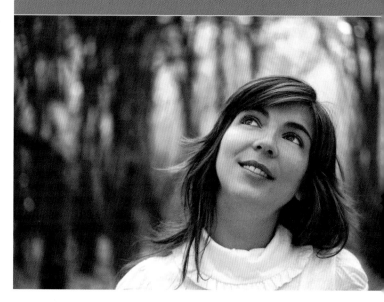

case, this will bring relief to the mind and often give health to the body.

Sympathy and tact will often prove a greater benefit to the sick than will the most skillful treatment given in a cold, indifferent way. When a physician comes to the sickbed with a listless, careless manner, looks at the afflicted one with little concern, by word or action giving the impression that the case is not one requiring much attention, and then leaves the patient to his own reflections, he has done that patient positive harm. The doubt and discouragement produced by his indifference will often counteract the good effect of the remedies he may prescribe. ~ The Ministry of Healing, pages 241, 244.

Another matter to keep in mind ...

We are in a world of suffering. Difficulty, trial, and sorrow await us all along the way to the heavenly home.

H 1. Be kind and gentle toward others.

But there are many who make life's burdens doubly heavy by continually anticipating trouble. If they meet with adversity or disappointment they think that everything is going to ruin, that theirs is the hardest lot of all, that they are surely coming to poverty. Thus they bring wretchedness upon themselves and cast a shadow upon all around them. Life itself becomes a burden to them. But it need not be so. It will take a determined effort to change the current of their thought. But the change can be made. Their happiness, both for this life and for the life to come, depends upon their fixing their minds upon cheerful things. Let them look away from the dark picture, which is imaginary, to the benefits which God has strewn in their pathway, and beyond these to the unseen and eternal.

For every trial, God has provided help. When Israel in the desert came to the bitter waters of Marah, Moses cried unto the Lord. The Lord did not provide some new remedy; He called attention to what was nearby. A shrub which He had created was to be cast into the fountain to make the water pure and sweet. When this was done, the people drank of the water and were refreshed. In every trial, if we seek Him, Christ will give us help. Our eyes will be opened to discern the healing promises recorded in His word. The Holy Spirit will teach us how to appropriate every blessing that will be an antidote to grief. For every bitter cup that is placed to our lips, we shall find a branch of healing.

We are not to let the future, with its hard problems, its unsatisfying prospects, make our hearts faint, our knees tremble, our hands hang down. "Let him take hold of My strength," says the Mighty One, "that he may make peace with Me; and he shall make peace with Me." Isaiah 27:5. Those who surrender their lives to His guidance and to His service will never be placed in a position for which He has not made provision. Whatever our situation, if we are doers of His word, we have a Guide to direct our way; whatever our perplexity, we have a sure Counselor; whatever our sorrow, bereavement, or loneliness, we have a sympathizing Friend.

If in our ignorance we make missteps, the Savior does not forsake us. We need never feel that we are alone. Angels are our companions. The Comforter that Christ promised to send in His name abides with us. In the way that leads to the City of God there are no difficulties which those who trust in Him may not overcome. There are no dangers which they may not escape. There is not a sorrow, not a grievance, not a human weakness, for which He has not provided a remedy.

None need abandon themselves to discouragement and despair. Satan may come to you with the cruel suggestion, "Yours is a hopeless case. You are irredeemable." But there is hope for you in Christ. God does not ask us to

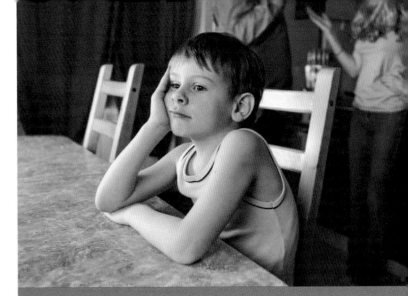

A troubled home life can cause a lot of stress on children and adults. Stress is a normal part of life, but we must deal with it appropriately, since too much stress can lead to physical problems such as: [4]

- Headaches
- Fatigue
- Sleep Problems
- Upset Stomach
  - Cramps, Constipation, Diarrhea
- Irritability
- Depression
- High Blood Pressure
- Abnormal Heartbeat (arrhythmia)
- Hardening of the Arteries (atherosclerosis)
- Heart Disease
- Heart Attack
- Heartburn
- Ulcers
- Irritable Bowel Syndrome
- Weight Gain or Loss
- Fertility Problems
- Flare-ups of Asthma or Arthritis
- Skin Problems such as Acne, Eczema, Psoriasis.

Read Habit #7, "Healthy Balance", to help with stress management. Protect your family and yourself from unnecessary ailments. Seek out professional help if necessary: your medical health provider, a counselor, clergy member etc.

overcome in our own strength. He asks us to come close to His side. Whatever difficulties we labor under, which weigh down soul and body, He waits to make us free.

He who took humanity upon Himself knows how to sympathize with the sufferings of humanity. Not only does Christ know every person, and the peculiar needs and trials of that person, but He knows all the circumstances that chafe and perplex the spirit. His hand is outstretched in pitying tenderness to every suffering child. Those who suffer most have most of His sympathy and pity. He is touched with the feeling of our infirmities, and He desires us to lay our perplexities and troubles at His feet and leave them there.

It is not wise to look to ourselves and study our emotions. If we do this, the enemy will present difficulties and temptations that weaken faith and destroy courage. To study our emotions closely and give way to our feelings is to entertain doubt and entangle ourselves in perplexity. We are to look away from self to Jesus.

When temptations assail you, when care, perplexity, and darkness seem to surround your soul, look to the place where you last saw the light. Rest in Christ's love and under His protecting care. When sin struggles for the mastery in the heart, when guilt oppresses the soul and burdens the conscience, when unbelief clouds the mind, remember that Christ's grace is sufficient to subdue sin and banish the darkness. Entering into communion with the Savior, we enter the region of peace. ~ The Ministry of Healing, pages 247-250.

When someone asks how you are feeling, do not try to think of something mournful to tell in order to gain sympathy. Do not talk of your lack of faith and your sorrows and sufferings. The tempter delights to hear such words. When talking on gloomy subjects, you are glorifying him. We are not to dwell on the great power of Satan to overcome us. Often we give ourselves into his hands by talking of his power. Let us talk instead of the great power of God to unite all our interests with His own. Tell of the matchless power of Christ, and speak of His glory. All heaven is

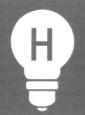

2. Let your thoughts dwell on the positive things of life rather than the difficulties.

interested in our salvation. The angels of God, thousands upon thousands, and ten thousand times ten thousand, are commissioned to minister to those who shall be heirs of salvation. They guard us against evil and press back the powers of darkness that are seeking our destruction. Have we not reason to be thankful every moment, thankful even when there are apparent difficulties in our pathway? ~ The Ministry of Healing, pages 253, 254.

DOCTOR SAYS

Your mind needs "exercise" just like your body does. Some ways you can "exercise" your mind are:

- Learning new things. For example:
  - Studying a new language
  - Learning how to play a musical instrument
  - Memorizing passages from the Bible
  - Developing the artistic side of yourself

- Focusing on the positive things of life rather than the negative
- Interacting with people
- Spending time in nature
- Generally speaking, things that are good for the body tend to be good for the brain and the mind.

- Choosing to be happy and joyful
- Laugh, smile, laugh, smile. Find humor in life, and don't forget to laugh and smile.
- Get professional counseling or help if you need to.

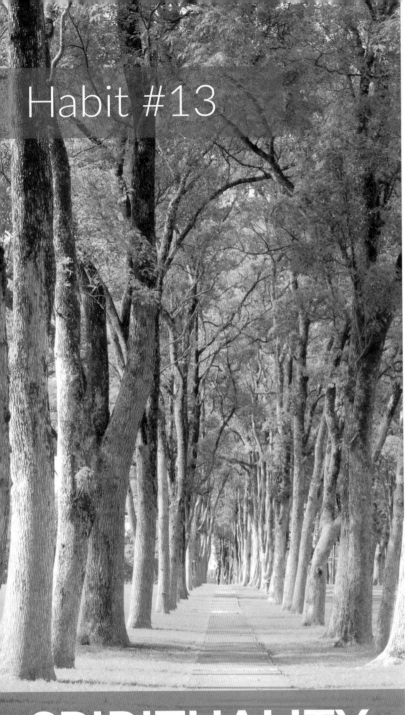

Habit #13

SPIRITUALITY

Jesus looked upon the distressed and heart-burdened, those whose hopes were blighted, and who with earthly joys were seeking to quiet the longing of the soul, and He invited all to find rest in Him. ~ The Ministry of Healing, page 71.

B ecause God's love is so great and so unfailing, the sick should be encouraged to trust in Him and be cheerful. ~ The Ministry of Healing, page 229.

The whole Bible is a revelation of the glory of God in Christ. Received, believed, obeyed, it is the great instrumentality in the transformation of character. It is the grand stimulus, the constraining force, that quickens the physical, mental, and spiritual powers, and directs the life into right channels. ~ The Ministry of Healing, page 458.

We are finding out more and more how intricately related each aspect of our health is to the other parts. Spiritual, mental, emotional, social, and physical health are all interrelated. In this chapter, we will be discussing more about spiritual health.

We believe that each person can and should choose what to believe in. This book will look at spirituality from a Christian perspective, since we are following the lifestyle habits of the Seventh-day Adventist Christians.

Although Henry and Anna claim Christianity as their choice of religion to express their spirituality, they do not participate in much of the Christian lifestyle. They rarely pray, they have a very dusty Bible that they hardly ever open, they rarely go to church, and although they would love to, they hardly ever are able to volunteer their time or money to help with outreach efforts. When asked the question, "Are you satisfied with your current spiritual life?" they both answered "No." They both want to have a stronger Christian walk.

So how do we develop a stronger walk with God?

Simply put, the essence of Christianity is to know Jesus Christ—to have a personal, trusting relationship with God. There is a deep peace to be experienced in being able to trust in a Higher Being that we believe knows what is best for us individually and has our best interests in mind.

But, how do we get to know Jesus Christ? How do we get to know God?

Many are the ways in which God is seeking to make Himself known to us and bring us into communion with Him. Nature speaks to our senses without ceasing. The open heart will be impressed with the love and glory of God as revealed through the works of His hands. **The listening ear can hear and understand the communications of God through the things of nature.** *The green fields, the lofty trees, the buds and flowers, the passing cloud, the falling rain, the babbling brook, the glories of the heavens, speak to our hearts, and invite us to become acquainted with Him who made them all.*

Our Savior bound up His precious lessons with the things of nature. The trees, the birds, the flowers of the valleys, the hills, the lakes, and the beautiful heavens, as well as the incidents and surroundings of daily life, were all linked with the words of truth, that His lessons might thus be often recalled to mind, even amid the busy cares of our life of toil.

God would have His children appreciate His works and delight in the simple, quiet beauty with which He has adorned our earthly home. He is a lover of the beautiful, and above all that is outwardly attractive He loves beauty of character; He would have us cultivate purity and simplicity, the quiet graces of the flowers.

If we will but listen, God's created works will teach us precious lessons of obedience and trust. From the stars that in their trackless courses through space follow from age to age their appointed path, down to the minutest atom, the things of nature obey the Creator's will. And God cares for everything and sustains everything that He has created. He who upholds the unnumbered worlds throughout immensity, at the same time cares for the wants of the little brown sparrow that sings its humble song without fear. When people go out to their daily toil, as when they engage in prayer; when they lie down at night, and when they rise in the morning; when the rich feast in their palaces, or when the poor gather their children around the scanty table, each is tenderly watched by the heavenly Father. No tears are shed that God does not notice. There is no smile that He does not mark.

If we would only fully believe this, all undue anxieties would be dismissed. Our lives would not be so filled with disappointment as now; for everything, whether great or small, would be left in the hands of God, who is not perplexed by the multiplicity of cares, or overwhelmed by their weight. We should then enjoy a rest of soul to which many have long been strangers.

As your senses delight in the attractive loveliness of the earth, think of the world that is to come, that shall never know the blight of sin and death; where the face of

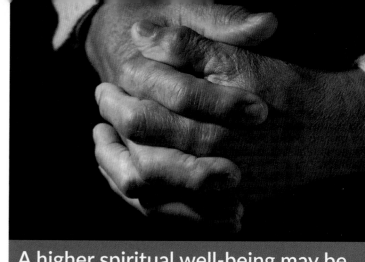

A higher spiritual well-being may be linked to:[1]

- -Less stress
- -Lower blood pressure
- -Lower risk of heart disease
- -Reduced depression

nature will no more wear the shadow of the curse. Let your imagination picture the home of the saved, and remember that it will be more glorious than your brightest imagination can portray. In the varied gifts of God in nature we see only the faintest gleaming of His glory. It is written, "Eye hath not seen, nor ear heard, neither have entered into the heart of man, the things which God hath prepared for them that love Him." 1 Corinthians 2:9.

The poet and the naturalist have many things to say about nature, but it is the Christian who enjoys the beauty of the earth with the highest appreciation, because he recognizes his Father's handiwork and perceives His love in flower and shrub and tree. No one can fully appreciate the significance of hill and vale, river and sea, who does not look upon them as an expression of God's love to mankind.

God speaks to us through His providential workings and through the influence of His Spirit upon the heart. *In our circumstances and surroundings, in the changes daily taking place around us, we may find precious lessons if our hearts are just open to discern them. The psalmist, tracing the work of God's providence, says, "The earth is full of the goodness of the Lord." "Whoso is wise, and will observe these things, even they shall*

GOD SPEAKS TO US THROUGH...
1. Nature   2. Providence   3. Influence of the Spirit   4. The Bible

Pray to God

"Prayer is the opening of the heart to God as to a friend... Prayer does not bring God down to us, but brings us up to Him." ~ Steps to Christ, page 93.

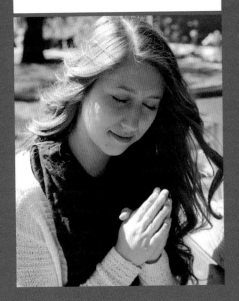

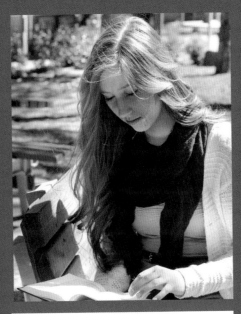

Share with someone

"No sooner does one come to Christ than there is born in his heart a desire to make known to others what a precious friend he has found in Jesus." ~ Steps to Christ, page 78.

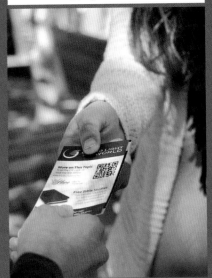

Study the Bible

"Fill the whole heart with the words of God. They are the living water, quenching your burning thirst." ~ Steps to Christ, page 88.

understand the loving-kindness of the Lord." Psalm 33:5; 107:43.

God speaks to us in His word. Here we have in clearer lines the revelation of His character, of His dealings with humanity, and the great work of redemption. Here is open before us the history of patriarchs and prophets and other holy men of old. They were men "subject to like passions as we are." James 5:17. We see how they struggled through discouragements like our own, how they fell under temptation as we have done, and yet took heart again and conquered through the grace of God; and, beholding, we are encouraged in our striving after righteousness. As we read of the precious experiences granted them, of the light and love and blessing it was theirs to enjoy, and of the work they accomplished through the grace given them, the spirit that inspired them kindles a flame of holy emulation in our hearts and a desire to be like them in character—like them to walk with God.

Jesus said of the Old Testament Scriptures—and how much more is it true of the New —"They are they which testify of Me," the Redeemer, Him in whom our hopes of eternal life are centered. John 5:39. Yes, the whole Bible tells of Christ. From the first record of creation—for "without Him was not anything made that was made—to the closing promise, "Behold, I come quickly," we are reading of His works and listening to His voice. John 1:3; Revelation 22:12. If you would become acquainted with the Savior, study the Holy Scriptures.

Fill the whole heart with the words of God. They are the living water, quenching your burning thirst. They are the living bread from heaven. Jesus declares, "Except ye eat the flesh of the Son of man, and drink His blood, ye have no life in you." And He explains Himself by saying, "The words that I speak unto you, they are spirit, and they are life." John 6:53, 63. Our bodies are built up from what we eat and drink; and as in the natural economy, so in the spiritual economy: it is what we meditate upon that will give tone and strength to our spiritual nature.

The theme of redemption is one that the angels desire to look into; it will be the science and the song of the redeemed throughout the ceaseless ages of eternity. Is it not worthy of careful thought and study now? The infinite mercy and love of Jesus, the sacrifice made in our behalf, call for the most serious and solemn reflection. We should dwell upon the character of our dear Redeemer and Intercessor. We should meditate upon the mission of Him who came to save His people from their sins. As we thus contemplate heavenly themes, our faith and love will grow stronger, and our prayers will be more and more acceptable to God, because they will be more and more mixed with faith and love. They will be intelligent and fervent. There will be more constant confidence in Jesus, and a daily, living experience in His power to save to the uttermost all that come unto God by Him.

As we meditate upon the perfections of the Savior, we shall desire to be wholly transformed and renewed in the image of His purity. There will be a hungering and thirsting of soul to become like Him whom we adore. The more our thoughts are upon Christ, the more we shall speak of Him to others and represent Him to the world.

The Bible was not written for the scholar alone; on the contrary, it was designed for the common people. The great truths necessary for salvation are made as clear as noonday; and none will mistake and lose their way except those who follow their own judgment instead of the plainly revealed will of God.

We should not take the testimony of anyone as to what the Scriptures teach, but should study the words of God for ourselves. If we allow others to do our thinking, we shall have crippled energies and contracted abilities. The noble powers of the mind may be so dwarfed by lack of exercise on themes worthy of their concentration as to lose their ability to grasp the deep meaning of the word of God. The mind will enlarge if it is employed in tracing out the relation of the subjects of the Bible, comparing scripture with scripture and spiritual things with spiritual.

There is nothing more calculated to strengthen the intellect than the study of the Scriptures. No other book is so potent to elevate the thoughts, to give vigor to the faculties, as the broad, ennobling truths of the Bible. If God's word were studied as it should be, people would have a breadth of mind, a nobility of character, and a stability of purpose rarely seen in these times.

But there is only a little benefit derived from a hasty reading of the Scriptures. One may read the whole Bible through and yet fail to see its beauty or comprehend its deep and hidden meaning. One passage studied until its significance is clear to the mind and its relation to the plan of salvation is evident, is of more value than the perusal of many chapters with no definite purpose in view and no positive instruction gained. Keep your Bible with you. As you have opportunity, read it; fix the texts in your memory. Even while you are walking the streets you may read a passage and meditate upon it, thus fixing it in the mind.

We cannot obtain wisdom without earnest attention and prayerful study. Some portions of Scripture are indeed too plain to be misunderstood, but there are others whose meaning does not lie on the surface to be seen

at a glance. Scripture must be compared with scripture. There must be careful research and prayerful reflection. And such study will be richly repaid. As the miner discovers veins of precious metal concealed beneath the surface of the earth, so will the person who perseveringly searches the word of God as for hid treasure find truths of the greatest value, which are concealed from the view of the careless seeker. The words of inspiration, pondered in the heart, will be as streams flowing from the fountain of life.

Never should the Bible be studied without prayer. Before opening its pages we should ask for the enlightenment of the Holy Spirit, and it will be given. When Nathanael came to Jesus, the Savior exclaimed, "Behold an Israelite indeed, in whom is no guile!" Nathanael said, "Whence knowest Thou me?" Jesus answered, "Before that Philip called thee, when thou wast under the fig tree, I saw thee." John 1:47, 48. And Jesus will see us also in the secret places of prayer if we will seek Him for light that we may know what is truth. Angels from the world of light will be with those who in humility of heart seek for divine guidance.

The Holy Spirit exalts and glorifies the Savior. It is His work to present Christ, the purity of His righteousness, and the great salvation that we have through Him. Jesus says, "He shall receive of Mine, and shall show it unto you." John 16:14. The Spirit of truth is the only effectual teacher of divine truth. How must God esteem the human race, since He gave His Son

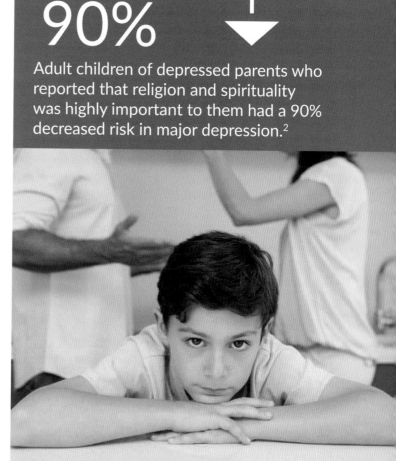

90% ⬇

Adult children of depressed parents who reported that religion and spirituality was highly important to them had a 90% decreased risk in major depression.[2]

to die for us and appoints His Spirit to be our teacher and continual guide! ~ Steps to Christ, pages 85-91.

Not only do we experience peace of mind in knowing Jesus as our Friend and Savior, but we also reap health benefits, as you saw previously.

Henry and Anna want to improve their spiritual life and prioritize this important aspect of their lives. Here are some changes that they can make:

- Pray individually and together as a couple.
- Read and study their Bible.
- Connect with other like-minded people.
- Connect with a Bible-believing church.
- Visit this website to locate a nearby Christian Church:
  - http://www.adventist.org/utility/find-a-church/

The improvement of our spiritual health is a journey throughout our lifetime. Developing a strong, trusting relationship with God does not happen overnight. Just like any other meaningful relationship in life takes time and effort, so it is with God. These simple steps will give you the foundation that you need to develop a meaningful relationship with God.

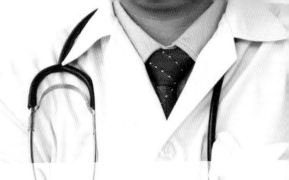

There are a number of things that contribute to our spiritual well-being. Here are just a few of them:

- Sincere prayer: just speak to God as you would to your most trusted friend!
- Reading and studying your Bible.
- Belonging to a church family.
- Sharing the love of God with others.

Try them today!

DOCTOR SAYS

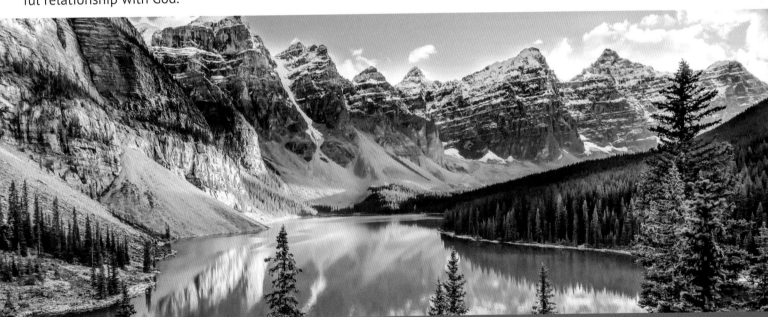

RESOURCES

Here is a list of websites you can access for resources on how to improve your spiritual health:

- amazingfacts.org
- glowonline.org
- 3abn.org
- llbn.tv
- itiswritten.com

TESTIMONIAL

Anthony

At just 20 years old, Anthony weighed 335 pounds, more than double his ideal body weight for his height and frame. He had tried to drown out his daily stresses with long hours of video games, cigarettes, and alcohol. He loved to snack on junk food all day long with heavily caffeinated energy drinks. His favorite thing to eat was a thick piece of medium-rare steak.

As his interest in spiritual things increased, his physical health improved as well.

One day, Anthony thought to himself, "I need to get healthier." He made a decision to stop drinking soda and replaced it with water. In just one week he lost ten lbs. Just a few months afterward, he started to gain an interest in his spiritual health as well. He began to attend a local Christian church. Not only did he grow healthier spiritually, but he also gained a valuable knowledge of healthy physical living from the Bible. He learned that our bodies are the temple of God, so we should do our best to take care of them. He also learned that God's ideal menu plan is plant-based. As his interest in spiritual things increased, his physical health improved as well.

Soon after, Anthony stopped eating pork and other unhealthful meats as outlined in the Bible in Leviticus 11. Eventually he was able to stop drinking alcohol and also stopped smoking. He stopped drinking the energy drinks and was even able to control his snacking addiction. Several months later, Anthony became a vegetarian, deciding that he wanted to try out God's ideal menu plan found in the Bible. He eventually replaced the dairy and eggs with other healthier alternatives.

Through his journey of "getting healthier," Anthony lost over 150 pounds and found more wholesome ways to meet his daily stresses. His newfound faith in God grew, and even his relationships with family and friends improved. Today, he actively serves as a teacher and speaker in sharing with others how they too can live happily and healthfully in Jesus.

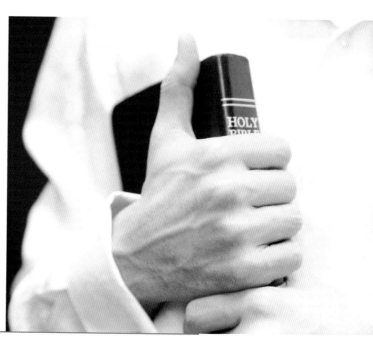

SERVICE

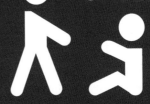

Remember that true joy can be found only in unselfish service. ~The Ministry of Healing, page 362.

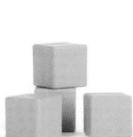

Good deeds are twice a blessing, benefiting both the giver and the receiver of the kindness. The consciousness of right-doing is one of the best medicines for diseased bodies and minds. When the mind is free and happy from a sense of duty well done and the satisfaction of giving happiness to others, the cheering, uplifting influence brings new life to the whole being. ~ The Ministry of Healing, page 257.

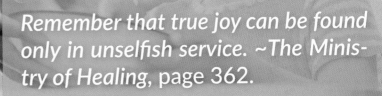

UNSELFISH SERVICE

May be linked to:
Lower Blood Pressure
and
Longer Lifespan

Studies are suggesting that people who give their time in unselfish service may have better physical health, evidenced in such things as lower blood pressure and a longer lifespan.[1]

Let the long-term sick, instead of constantly requiring sympathy, seek to impart it. Let the burden of your own weakness and sorrow and pain be cast upon the compassionate Savior. Open your heart to His love, and let it flow out to others. Remember that all have trials hard to bear, temptations hard to resist, and you may do something to lighten these burdens. Express gratitude for the blessings you have; show appreciation of the at-

tentions you receive. Keep the heart full of the precious promises of God, that you may bring forth from this treasure, words that will be a comfort and strength to others. This will surround you with an atmosphere that will be helpful and uplifting. Let it be your aim to bless those around you, and you will find ways of being helpful, both to the members of your own family and to others.

If those who are suffering from ill-health would forget self in their interest for others; if they would fulfill the Lord's command to minister to those more needy than themselves, they would realize the truthfulness of the prophetic promise, "Then shall thy light break forth as the morning, and thine health shall spring forth speedily." ~ The Ministry of Healing, pages 257, 258.

VOLUNTEERISM AMONG OLDER ADULTS HAS BEEN LINKED TO: [2]

- Greater life satisfaction
- More purpose in life
- Greater self-esteem
- Increased personal control
- Fewer depressive symptoms

"In all things I have shown you that by working hard in this way we must help the weak and remember the words of the Lord Jesus, how he himself said, 'It is more blessed to give than to receive.'"—Acts 20:35 ESV

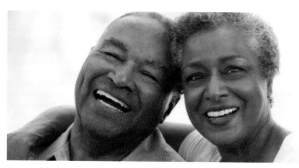

Although there are various known health benefits from volunteering and helping others, that should not be our motivation to help others. Yes, studies have indicated that helping others could help with hypertension, depression, increased lifespan, and other matters, but more importantly we are called to help and build each other up.

ROMANS 12:10
"Be kindly affectioned one to another with brotherly love; in honour preferring one another." (KJV)

GALATIANS 6:2
"Bear one another's burdens, and so fulfill the law of Christ." (ESV)

JOHN 13:34
"A new commandment I give unto you, that ye love one another; as I have loved you, that ye also love one another." (KJV)

HEBREWS 13:1
"Let brotherly love continue." (KJV)

PROVERBS 11:25
"Whoever brings blessing will be enriched, and one who waters will himself be watered." (ESV)

PHILIPPIANS 2:3, 4
"Let nothing be done through selfish ambition or conceit, but in lowliness of mind let each esteem others better than himself. Let each of you look out not only for his own interests, but also for the interests of others." (NKJV)

Helping in an area that matches your skill set and personality can make volunteering very enjoyable and something that you look forward to. Contact the local church pastor or other nonprofit community organizations for opportunities to volunteer and give back to the community.

It is part of the longevity lifestyle of Seventh-day Adventists to live for something bigger than themselves. They take part in many volunteer efforts to help those in need around them. It is part of the mission of genuine Christians to help those in need, to share with them the love of Jesus Christ. The Bible says in Proverbs 29:18: "Where there is no vision, the people perish." It seems that the people who have the deep abiding joy in their lives are living for something bigger than themselves. It seems that they have a bigger purpose, a bigger vision in life than to just please themselves. They tend to have a mission for helping and serving, whether it is for other people, the earth, or working for God.

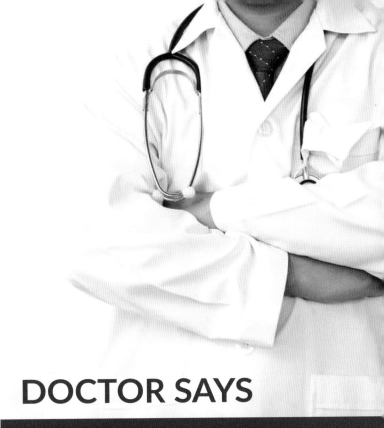

DOCTOR SAYS

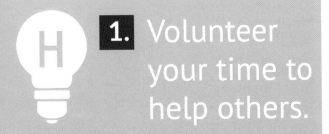

1. Volunteer your time to help others.

Help others. Visit the sick. Feed the hungry. Be a friend. Love others. Have a purpose and goal in life. Get to know Jesus Christ.

"For I was hungry and you gave me food, I was thirsty and you gave me drink, I was a stranger and you welcomed me, I was naked and you clothed me, I was sick and you visited me, I was in prison and you came to me.' Then the righteous will answer him, saying, 'Lord, when did we see you hungry and feed you, or thirsty and give you drink? And when did we see you a stranger and welcome you, or naked and clothe you? And when did we see you sick or in prison and visit you?' And the King will answer them, 'Truly, I say to you, as you did it to one of the least of these my brothers, you did it to me.'"—Matthew 25:35-40 ESV

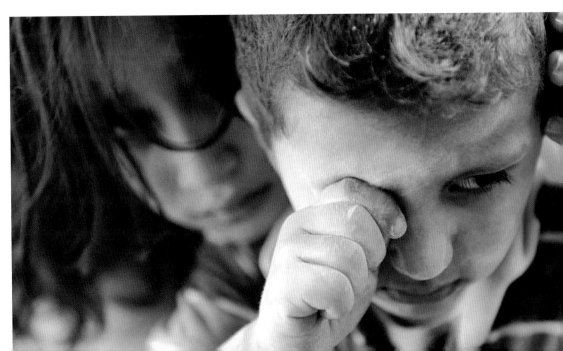

Epilogue

If Henry and Anna apply the habits presented in this book, their health could dramatically improve. Anna could shed the extra weight that she has been wanting to lose for years. Henry doesn't have to live in fear of dying from a heart attack like his father did. They could have more family time and develop better relationships with others. Henry could start enjoying the great outdoors like he used to. Anna doesn't have to be depressed. They could have a strong spiritual life. They could have the time and the energy to give back to their community and enjoy life together. Five to ten years from now, if they practice the habits in this book, their lives could be drastically different.

What about you? What would happen if you followed these habits that heal? How would your life look five to ten years from now? And if you don't follow these habits, how will your life look five to ten years down the road? How will your family be affected? Your work? Your life goals?

So, what will you do now? The choice is yours.

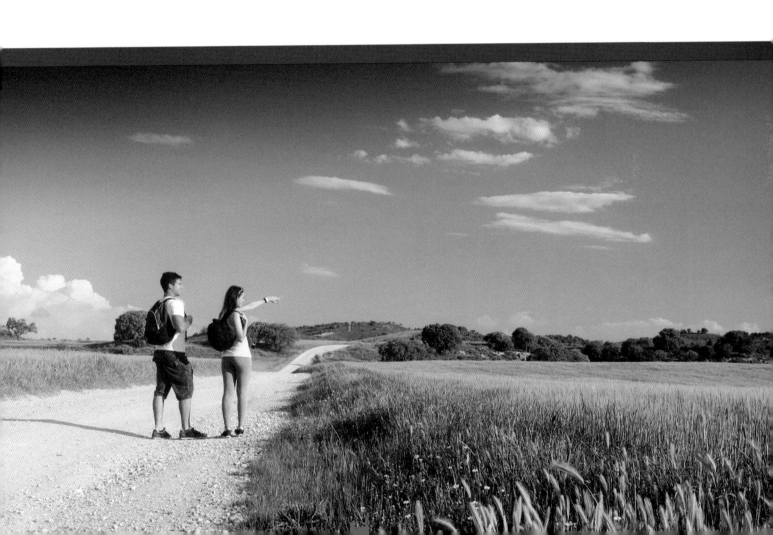

Citations

Habit #1 The Power of Choice

1. Treating Depression. (2014, August 14). Retrieved March 6, 2015, from http://www.webmd.com/depression/takingfirststep-healthcareprovidersstreatingdepres sionmedref

Habit #2 Water, the Elixir of Life

1. Mayo Clinic Staff. (2014, September 5). Nutrition and Healthy Eating. Retrieved March 4, 2015, from http://www.mayoclinic. org/healthyliving/nutritionandhealthyeating/indepth/water/art 20044256

2. Blackmer, S. (2012). Celebrating Liquids. In *Celebrations: Living Life to the Fullest*. (p. 56). Silver Spring, MD: Health Ministries Dept.

3. Mayo Clinic Staff. (2014, September 5). Nutrition and Healthy Eating. Retrieved March 4, 2015, from http://www.mayoclinic. org/healthyliving/nutritionandhealthyeating/indepth/water/art 20044256

4. Lieberson, A. (2004, November 8). How long can a person survive without food? Retrieved February 28, 2015 from http://www.scientificamerican.com/article/howlongcanapersonsur/.

5. Negoianu, D., & Goldfarb, S. (2008). Just Add Water. (10466673/19061041). Retrieved February 28, 2015, from the Journal of the American Society of Nephrology.

6. Mayo Clinic Staff. (2014, September 5). Nutrition and Healthy Eating. Retrieved March 4, 2015, from http://www.mayoclinic. org/healthyliving/nutritionandhealthyeating/indepth/water/art 20044256

7. Mayo Clinic Staff. (2014, September 5). Nutrition and Healthy Eating. Retrieved March 4, 2015, from http://www.mayoclinic. org/healthyliving/nutritionandhealthyeating/indepth/water/art 20044256

8. Ronbinson, J. (2014, October 6.). Constipation Symptoms, Causes, and Diagnosis. Retrieved March 25, 2015, from http://www.webmd.com/digestivedisorders/digestivediseases-constipation

9. Blackmer, S. (2012). Celebrating Liquids. In *Celebrations: Living life to the Fullest*. (p. 63). Silver Spring, MD.: Health Ministries Dept.

10. Malik, A., Akram, Y., Shetty, S., Malik, S., & Njike, V. (2014). Impact of SugarSweetened Beverages on Blood Pressure. 1574-1580. Retrieved December 2, 2014, from The American Journal of Cardiology.

11. Mcneilus, M. (2010). The Contrast Bath. *In Nature's Healing Way* (pp. 3639). Decatur, Georgia: Home Health Education Services.

12. Blackmer, S. (2012). Celebrating Liquids. In *Celebrations: Living life to the Fullest.* (p. 65). Silver Spring, MD.: Health Min. Dept.

Habit #3 No Exercise, Know Sickness

1. Buchner, D., Bishop, J., Brown, D., Fulton, J., Galuska, D., Gilchrist, J., . . . Rodgers, A. (2008). Physical Activity Has Many Health Benefits. In *2008 Physical Activities Guidelines for Americans* (p. 9). U.S. Department of Health and Human Services

2. Chobotar, T. (2013). Immediate Benefits. In *Activity Supercharges Your Life* (Vol. 4 CREATION Health Life Guide, p. 80). Maitland, Florida: Florida Hospital Publishing

3 . Powerful Reasons to Exercise. (2014 , March 1) . Retrieved February 20 , 2015, from h ttp://www.emedexpert.com/tips/exercise.shtml

4. Powerful Reasons to Exercise. (2014, March 1). Retrieved February 20, 2015, from h ttp://www.emedexpert.com/tips/exercise.shtml

5. Powerful Reasons to Exercise. (2014, March 1). Retrieved February 20, 2015, from http://www.emedexpert.com/tips/exercise.shtml

6. Powerful Reasons to Exercise. (2014, March 1). Retrieved February 20, 2015, from h ttp://www.emedexpert.com/tips/exercise.shtml

7. Powerful Reasons to Exercise. (2014, March 1). Retrieved February 20, 2015, from h ttp://www.emedexpert.com/tips/exercise.shtml

8. Powerful Reasons to Exercise. (2014, March 1). Retrieved February 20, 2015, from h ttp://www.emedexpert.com/tips/exercise.shtml

9. Park, A. (2012, July 18). Lack of Exercise as Deadly as Smoking, Study Finds. *TIME Magazine*, retrieved from http://healthland.time.com/2012/07/18/lackofexerciseasdeadlyassmokingstudyfinds/

Habit #4 Rest is Best

1. Why Is Sleep Important? (2012, February 22). Retrieved March 1, 2015, from h ttp://www.nhlbi.nih.gov/health/healthtopics/topics/sdd/why

2. What Happens When You Sleep? (n.d.). Retrieved March 1, 2015, from http://sleepfoundation.org/howsleepworks/what-happenswhenyousleep

3. Brain Basics: Understanding Sleep. (2014, July 25). Retrieved February 9, 2015, from http://www.ninds.nih.gov/disorders/brain_basics/understanding_sleep.htm

4. Why Is Sleep Important? (2012, February 22). Retrieved March 1, 2015, from http://www.nhlbi.nih.gov/health/healthtopics/topics/sdd/why

5. Sleep and Disease Risk. (2007, December 18). Retrieved March 3, 2015, from http://healthysleep.med.harvard.edu/healthy/matters/consequences/sleepanddiseaserisk

6. Sleep and Disease Risk. (2007, December 18). Retrieved March 3, 2015, from http://healthysleep.med.harvard.edu/healthy/matters/consequences/sleepanddiseaserisk

7. Griffin, R. (2011, December 27). 9 Surprising Reasons to Get More Sleep. Retrieved March 5, 2015, from http://www.webmd.com/sleepdisorders/features/9reasonstosleepmore?page=3

8. Why Is Sleep Important? (2012, February 22). Retrieved March 1, 2015, from http://www.nhlbi.nih.gov/health/healthtopics/topics/sdd/why.

9. Sleep and Disease Risk. (2007, December 18). Retrieved March 3, 2015, from http://healthysleep.med.harvard.edu/healthy/matters/consequences/sleepanddiseaserisk

10. Why Is Sleep Important? (2012, February 22). Retrieved March 1, 2015, from http://www.nhlbi.nih.gov/health/healthtopics/topics/sdd/why.

11. Mann, D., Smith, M., (2010, January 19). Lack of Sleep and the Immune System. Retrieved February 6, 2015, from http://www.webmd.com/sleepdisorders/excessivesleepiness10/immune-systemlackof sleep

12. Why Is Sleep Important? (2012, February 22). Retrieved March 1, 2015, from http://www.nhlbi.nih.gov/health/healthtopics/topics/sdd/why.

13. Griffin, R., Chang, L. (2011, December 27). 9 Surprising Reasons to Get More Sleep. Retrieved March 5, 2015, from http://www.webmd.com/sleepdisorders/features/9reasonstosleepmore?page=3

14. Why Is Sleep Important? (2012, February 22). Retrieved March 1, 2015, from http://www.nhlbi.nih.gov/health/healthtopics/topics/sdd/why

15. Griffin, R. (2011, December 27). 9 Surprising Reasons to Get More Sleep. Retrieved March 5, 2015, from http://www.webmd.com/sleepdisorders/features/9reasonstosleepmore?page=3k

16. Griffin, R. (2011, December 27). 9 Surprising Reasons to Get More Sleep. Retrieved March 5, 2015, from http://www.webmd.com/sleepdisorders/features/9reasonstosleepmore?page=3

17. National Institute of Neurological Disorders and Stroke (NINDS) (n.d.). Retrieved February 28, 2015, from h ttp://www.ninds.nih.gov/ 18. Twery, M. (2014, December 29). Why is Sleep Important? Retrieved April 9, 2015, from http://www.hhs.gov/blog/2014/12/29/whysleepimportant.html

Habit #5 The Effects of Your Environment

1. Louv, R. (2011). Nature Neurons. In *The Nature Principle* (pp. 3334). New York, New York: Algonquin Books of Chapel Hill.

2. Johnson, K. (2004). Valuing Nature. In *You Were Made for a Garden* (Vol.3, CREATION Health Life Guide, p. 22). Maitland, Florida: Florida Hospital Publishing.

3. Gardening for Health. (2000, October 30). Retrieved February 20, 2015, from http://www.webmd.com/healthyaging/features/gardeninghealth

4 . Johnson , K . (2004). Valuing Nature. In *You Were Made for a Garden* (Vol. 3, CREATION Health Life Guide, p. 32). Maitland, Florida: Florida Hospital Publishing.

5. Dunkin, M. (2010, September 12). 6 Surprisingly Dirty Places in Your Home. Retrieved February 21, 2015, from http://www.webmd.com/women/homehealthandsafety9/placesgermshide

6. Dunkin, M. (2010, September 12). 6 Surprisingly Dirty Places in Your Home. Retrieved February 21, 2015, from http://www.webmd.com/women/homehealthandsafety9/placesgermshide

7. Dunkin, M. (2010, September 12). 6 Surprisingly Dirty Places in Your Home. Retrieved February 21, 2015, from http://www.webmd.com/women/homehealthandsafety9/placesgermshide

8. Dunkin, M. (2010, September 12). 6 Surprisingly Dirty Places in Your Home. Retrieved February 21, 2015, from http://www.webmd.com/women/homehealthandsafety9/placesgermshide

9. Dunkin, M. (2010, September 12). 6 Surprisingly Dirty Places in Your Home. Retrieved February 21, 2015, from http://www.webmd.com/women/homehealthandsafety9/placesgermshide

10. Dunkin, M. (2010, September 12). 6 Surprisingly Dirty Places in Your Home. Retrieved February 21, 2015, from http://www.webmd.com/women/homehealthandsafety9/placesgermshide

11. Dunkin, M. (2010, September 12). 6 Surprisingly Dirty Places in Your Home. Retrieved February 21, 2015, from http://www.webmd.com/women/homehealthandsafety9/placesgermshide

12. Dunkin, M. (2010, September 12). 6 Surprisingly Dirty Places in Your Home. Retrieved February 21, 2015, from http://www.webmd.com/women/homehealthandsafety9/placesgermshide

13. Dunkin, M. (2010, September 12). 6 Surprisingly Dirty Places in Your Home. Retrieved February 21, 2015, from http://www.webmd.com/women/homehealthandsafety9/placesgermshide

14. Dunkin, M. (2010, September 12). 6 Surprisingly Dirty Places in Your Home. Retrieved February 21, 2015, from http://www.webmd.com/women/homehealthandsafety9/placesgermshide

15. Dunkin, M. (2010, September 12). 6 Surprisingly Dirty Places in Your Home. Retrieved February 21, 2015, from http://www.webmd.com/women/homehealthandsafety9/placesgermshide

16. Dunkin, M. (2010, September 12). 6 Surprisingly Dirty Places in Your Home. Retrieved February 21, 2015, from http://www.webmd.com/women/homehealthandsafety9/placesgermshide

Habit #6 Fresh Air & Sunlight

1. How Your Body Uses Oxygen. (2013, March 5). Retrieved February 8, 2015, from https://patienteducation.osumc.edu/Documents/howbodyoxygen.pdf

2. Dean, L. (2005). Blood and the Cells it Contains. In *Blood Groups and Red Cell Antigens*. Bethesda, MD: National Center for Biotechnology Information. R etrieved March 5, 2015, from h ttp://www.ncbi.nlm.nih.gov/books/NBK2263/

3. Deep Breathing: StepbyStep Stress Relief. (2013, June 18). Retrieved March 3, 2015, from http://www.webmd.com/parenting/raisingfitkids/recharge/howtodeepbreathe

4. Deep Breathing: StepbyStep Stress Relief. (2013, June 18). Retrieved March 3, 2015, from http://www.webmd.com/parenting/raisingfitkids/recharge/howtodeepbreathe

5. Masamoto, K., & Tanishita K. (2009) Oxygen transport in brain tissue. National Center for Biotechnology Information. Retrieved March 3, 2015, from National Center Biotechnology Information from h ttp:www/ncbi.nlm.nih.gov/pubmed/19640134

6. Neuroscience For Kids. (n.d.). Retrieved March 3, 2015, from http://faculty.washington.edu/chudler/vessel.html

7. Satish, U., Mendell, M., Krishnamurthy, S., Toshifumi, H., Sullivan, D., Siegfried, S., & Fisk, W. (2012). Effects of CO2 on decision making performance. Environmental Health Perspectives, 120(12), 16711677. Retrieved March 3, 2015, from Environmental Health Perspectives.

8. Vitamin D: Fact Sheet for Health Professionals (2014, November 10). Retrieved March 4, 2015, from h ttp://ods.od.nih.gov/factsheets/VitaminDHealthProfessional/

9. Kotz, D. (2008, June 24). Host of Health Benefits Attributed to Sunlight. Retrieved March 1, 2015, from http://health.usnews.com/healthnews/familyhealth/articles/2008/06/24/hostofhealthbe nefitsattributedtosunlight

10. Mead, M. (2008, May). Benefits of Sunlight A Bright Spot for Human Health. Environmental Health Perspectives, 116 (4), 161-167. Retrieved February 23, 2015 from http://www.ncbi.nlm.nih.gov/pmc/articles/PMC2290997/.

11. Mead, M. (2008, May). Benefits of Sunlight A Bright Spot for Human Health. Environmental Health Perspectives, 116 (4), 161-167. Retrieved February 23, 2015 from http://www.ncbi.nlm.nih.gov/pmc/articles/PMC2290997/.

12. Kotz, D. (2008, June 24). Host of Health Benefits Attributed to Sunlight. Retrieved March 1, 2015, from http://health.usnews.com/healthnews/familyhealth/articles/2008/06/24/hostofhealthbe nefitsattributedtosunlight

13. Kotz, D. (2008, June 24). Host of Health Benefits Attributed to Sunlight. Retrieved March 1, 2015, from http://health.usnews.com/healthnews/familyhealth/articles/2008/06/24/hostofhealthbe nefitsattributedtosunlight

14. Melatonin for Sleep: Hormone and Supplement Effects on Sleep. (2012, June 20). Retrieved February 4, 2015, from h ttp://www.webmd.com/sleepdisorders/tc/melatoninoverview

15. Mayo Clinic Staff (2014, October 29). Diseases and Conditions: Rheumatoid Arthritis. Retrieved January 10, 2015, from http://www.mayoclinic.org/diseasesconditions/rheumatoidarthritis/basics/definition/CO N20014868

16. Arkema, E., Hart, J., Bertrand, K., Laden, F., Grodstein, F., Rosner, Bernard, R., Karlson, E., & Costenbader, K. (2013). Exposure to ultravioletB and risk of developing rheumatoid arthritis among women in the Nurses' Health Study. National Institute of Health, 506511. Retrieved December 20, 2014, from National Institute of Health.

17. Kotz, D. (2008, June 24). Host of Health Benefits Attributed to Sunlight. Retrieved March 1, 2015, from http://health.usnews.com/healthnews/familyhealth/articles/2008/06/24/hostofhealthbe nefitsattributedtosunlight

18. Riemersmavan der Lek, R., Swaab, D., Twisk, J., Hol, E., Hoogendijk, W., Van Someren, E.(2008). Effect of Bright Light and Melatonin on Cognitive and Noncognitive Function in Elderly Residents of Group Care Facillities: A Randomized Controlled Trial. 10(1001), 26422655. Retrieved March 20, 2015 from http://www.ncbi.nlm.nih.gov/pubmed/18544724.

Habit #7 Healthy Balance

1. Anderson, A. (2013, July 26). WorkLife Balance: 5 Ways To Turn It From The Ultimate Oxymoron Into A Real Plan. Retrieved March 1, 2015, from http://www.forbes.com/fdc/welcome_mjx.shtml

2. Uscher, J. (2013, March 28). 5 Tips for Better Work Life Balance. Retrieved March 9, 2015, from h ttp://www.webmd.com/healthinsurance/protecthealth13/balancelife?page=1

Habit #8 Eat to Live

1. Mekary, R., Giovannucci, E., Willett, W., Van Dam, R., & Hu, F. (2012). Eating patterns and type 2 diabetes risk in men: Breakfast omission, eating frequency, and snacking. American Journal of Clinical Nutrition, 11829. Retrieved January 3, 2015, from http://www.ncbi.nlm.nih.gov/pubmed/22456660

2. Mekary, R., Giovannucci, E., Willett, W., Van Dam, R., & Hu, F. (2012). Eating patterns and type 2 diabetes risk in men: Breakfast omission, eating frequency, and snacking. American Journal of Clinical Nutrition, 1189. Retrieved January 3, 2015, from http://www.ncbi.nlm.nih.gov/pubmed/22456660

Habit #9 Vegucate

1. McEvoy, C., Temple, N., & Woodside, J. (2012). Vegetarian diets, low meats diets and health: A review. Public Health Nutrition, 1 5 (12), 22882288. Retrieved February 3, 2015, from Cambridge Journals Online.

2. McEvoy, C., Temple, N., & Woodside, J. (2012). Vegetarian diets, low meats diets and health: A review. Public Health Nutrition, 1 5 (12), 22882288. Retrieved February 3, 2015, from Cambridge Journals Online.

3. Tonstad, S., Stewart, K., Oda, K., Batech, M., Herring, R., & Fraser, G. (2011). Vegetarian diets and incidence of diabetes in the Adventist Health Study2. Nutrition, Metabolism and Cardiovascular Diseases, 23(4), 292292.

4. Meat Consumption and Cancer Risk. (n.d.). Retrieved February 2, 2015, from http://www.pcrm.org/health/cancerresources/dietcancer/facts/meatconsumptionandca ncerrisk

5. Meat Consumption and Cancer Risk. (n.d.). Retrieved February 2, 2015, from http://www.pcrm.org/health/cancerresources/dietcancer/facts/meatconsumptionandca ncerrisk

6. Meat Consumption and Cancer Risk. (n.d.). Retrieved February 2, 2015, from http://www.pcrm.org/health/cancerresources/dietcancer/facts/meatconsumptionandca ncerrisk

7. Meat Consumption and Cancer Risk. (n.d.). Retrieved February 2, 2015, from http://www.pcrm.org/health/cancerresources/dietcancer/facts/meatconsumptionandcancerrisk

8. Orlich, M., Signh, P., Sabate, J., JaceldoSeigl, K., Fran, J., Knutsen, S., . . . Fraser, G. (2013). Vegetarian Dietary Patterns and Morality in Adventist Health Study 2. JAMA Intern Med, 173(13), 12301231.

9. Craig, W. (2009) Health Effects of Vegan Diets. R etrieved February 5, 2015, from A merican Journal of Clinical Nutrition, 1627S1633S

10. Tuso, P., Ismail, M., Ha, B., & Bartolotto, C. (n.d.). Nutritional Update for Physicians: PlantBased Diets. Retrieved January 17, 2015, from The Permanente Journal, 6166

11. Stoppler, M., Davis, C. (2014, June 18). Mad Cow Disease and Variant CreutzfeldtJakob Disease. Retrieved March 3, 2015, from http://www.emedicinehealth.com/mad_cow_disease_and_cariant_creutzfeldtjakob/articl e_em.htm

12. Salmonella (2015, March 9). Retrieved March 21, 2015, from http://www.cdc.gov/salmonella/general/

13. Salmonella Poisoning (Salmonellosis) Symptoms, Causes, Treatment. (2012, October 12). Retrieved from http://www.webmd.com/foodrecipes/foodpoisoning/salmonellosistopicoverview

14. Avila, J. (2012, March 7). 70 Percent of Ground Beef at Supermarkets Contains 'Pink Slime' ABC News. Retrieved February 27, 2015, from http://abcnews.go.com/blogs/headlines/2012/03/70-percentofgroundbeefatsupermarketscontainspinkslime/

15. Kearns, R., & Chang, MD, L. (2012, March 27). 'Pink Slime' Maker Cuts Down Production. Retrieved January 31, 2015, from http://www.webmd.com/foodrecipes/20120327/pinkslime-makercutsdownproduction

16. What's in That Pork? (2013, January 1). Retrieved February 10, 2015, from http://www.consumerreports.org/cro/maga-zine/2013/01/whatsinthatpor k/index.htm

17. Benefits of Fish. (2009, July 9). Retrieved February 10, 2015, from http://www.consumerreports.org/cro/2012/08/thebenefits-andrisksofeatingfish/index.htm

18. Weiss, K. (2002, December 9). Fish Farms Become Feedlots of the Sea. *LA Times*. Retrieved February 1, 2015, from http://www.latimes.com/nation/lamesalmon9dec09story.html#page=1

19. Benefits of Fish. (2009, July 9). Retrieved February 10, 2015, from http://www.consumerreports.org/cro/2012/08/thebenefits-andrisksofeatin gfish/index.htm

20. Norris, J. (2014, April 1). Omega3 Fatty Acid Recommenda-tions for Vegetarians. Retrieved February 10, 2015, from http://www.veganhealth.org/articles/omega3

21. K im, B., Laestadius, L., Lawrence, R., Martin, R., McKenzie, S., Nachman, K., . . . Truant, P. (n.d.). The Pew Commission on Indus-trial Farm Animal Production. *Putting Meat on the Table: Industrial Farm Animal Production in America*

22. Ending Factory Farming. (n.d.). Retrieved February 10, 2015, from http://www.farmforward.com/farmingforward/factory-farming

23. Birds on Factory Farms. ASPCA. (n.d.). Retrieved February 10, 2015, from https://www.aspca.org/fightcruelty/farmanimal-cruelty/birdsfactoryfarms

24. Cows on Factory Farms. ASPCA. (n.d.) Retrieved February 10, 2015, from https://www.aspca.org/fightcruelty/farmanimal-cruelty/cowsfactoryfarms

25. Pigs on Factory Farms. ASPCA. (n.d.) Retrieved February 20, 2015, from https://www.aspca.org/fightcruelty/farmanimal-cruelty/pigsfactoryfarms

26. Weiss, K. (2002, December 9). Fish Farms Become Feedlots of the Sea. *LA Times*. Retrieved February 1, 2015, from http://www.latimes.com/nation/lamesalmon9dec09story.html#page=1

27. Craig, W., & Mangels, A. (2009). Position of the American Di-etetic Association: Vegetarian diets. Journal of American Dietetic Association, 109(7), 126682. Retrieved from ncbi.nim.nih.gov

Habit #10 *Abstaining From The Deadly Three*

1. Evert, A. (2013, April 30). Caffeine in the Diet. Retrieved Feb-ruary 18, 2015, from http://www.nlm.nih.gov/medlineplus/ency/article/002445.htm

2. Evert, A. (2013, April 30). Caffeine in the Diet. Retrieved Feb-ruary 18, 2015, from http://www.nlm.nih.gov/medlineplus/ency/article/002445.htm

3. Vlachopoulos, C., Hirata, K., Stefanadis, C., Toutouzas, P., & O'Rourke, M. (2003, January). Caffeine Increases Aortic Stiffness in Hypertensive Patients 16 (1), 6366. Retrieved February 19, 2015, from American Journal of Hypertension

4. Klein, T. (n.d.). Energy Drinks Raise Resting Blood Pres-sure, Dramatic In those Not Used to Caffeine. Retrieved February 19, 2015, from http://newsnetwork.mayoclinic.org/discussion/energydrinksraiserestingbloodpressure witheffectmostdramaticinthosenotusedtocaffeinem/

5. Scher, A., Stewart, W., & Lipton, R. (2004). Caffeine as a Risk Factor for Chronic Daily Headache. Retrieved February 21, 2015, from http://neurology.org/content/63/11/2022.short

6. McMillin, A. (2011, June 1). School of Medicine Researcher Finds Link Between Caffeine Consumption and Female Infer-tility. Retrieved March 5, 2015, from http://unr.edu/nevada-today/news/2011/schoolofmedicineresearcherfindslinkbetwee ncaffeineconsumptionandfemaleinfertility

7. Lane, J., Barkauskas, C., Surwit, R., & Feinglos, M. (2004) Caffeine Impairs Glucose Metabolism in Type 2 Diabetes 27(8). Retrieved February 15, 2015, from The American Diabetes Asso-ciation

8. F aubion, S., Sood, R., Thielen, J., Shuster, L. (2015, February). Caffeine and Menopausal Symptoms: What is the Association? Retrieved March 11,2015, from http://www.ncbi.nlm.nih.gov/m/pubmed/25051286/

9. Keast, R., Swinburn, B., Sayompark, D., Whitelock S., Riddell, L. (2014) Caffeine Increases SugarSweetened Beverage Consump-tion in a FreeLiving Population: a Randomised Controlled Trial. Retrieved February 13, 2015, from British Journal of Nutrition

10. Health Effects of Secondhand Smoke. Center for Disease Control. (n.d.) Retrieved February 9, 2015, from http://www.cdc.gov/tobacco/data_statistics/fact_sheets/secondhad_smoke/heath_effects/

11. Health Effects of Secondhand Smoke. Center for Disease Control. (n.d.) Retrieved February 9, 2015, from http://www.cdc.gov/tobacco/data_statistics/fact_sheets/secondhad_smoke/heath_effects/

12. Health Effects of Secondhand Smoke. Center for Disease Control. (n.d.) Retrieved February 9, 2015, from http://www.cdc.gov/tobacco/data_statistics/fact_sheets/secondhad_smoke/heath_effects/

13. Health Effects of Cigarette Smoking. Center for Disease Control. (n.d.) Retrieved February 9, 2015 from http://www.cdc.gov/tobacco/data_statistics/fact_sheets/health_effects/effects_cig_smokin g/

14. Health Effects of Cigarette Smoking. Center for Disease Control. (n.d.) Retrieved February 9, 2015 from http://www.cdc.gov/tobacco/data_statistics/fact_sheets/health_effects/effects_cig_smokin g/

15. Health Effects of Cigarette Smoking. Center for Disease Control. (n.d.) Retrieved February 9, 2015 from http://www.cdc.gov/tobacco/data_statistics/fact_sheets/health_effects/effects_cig_smokin g/

16. Health Effects of Cigarette Smoking. Center for Disease Control. (n.d.) Retrieved February 9, 2015 from http://www.cdc.gov/tobacco/data_statistics/fact_sheets/health_effects/effects_cig_smokin g/

17. Fact Sheets Alcohol Use and Your Health. Center for Disease Control. (n.d.) Retrieved February 17, 2015, from h ttp://www.cdc.gov/alcohol/factsheets/alcoholuse.htm

18. Data, Trends and Maps. Center for Disease Control. (2014) Retrieved February 9, 2015, from http://nccd.cdc.gov/DHD-SP_DTM/

19. FAQ. National Council on Alcoholism and Drug Dependence. (n.d.) Retrieved March 11, 2015, from h ttp://ncadd.org/learn-aboutalcoholfaqsfacts

20. Fact Sheets Alcohol Use and Your Health. Centers for Disease Control. (n.d.) Retrieved February 17, 2015, from h ttp://www.cdc.gov/alcohol/factsheets/alcoholuse.htm

21. Rehm, J., (2011). The Risks Associated With Alcohol Use and Alcoholism. Retrieved February 9, 2015, from Alcohol Research & Health, Volume 34, Number 2

22. Alcohol and Pregnancy. National Institutes of Health. (n.d.) Retrieved March 3, 2015, from http://www.nlm.nih.gov/medline-plus/ency/article/007454.htm

Habit #11 Interpersonal Relationships

1. Marital Stress Worsens Prognosis in Women With Coronary Heart Disease. (2000, December 20). Retrieved February 18, 2015, from http://jama.jamanetwork.com/article.aspx? articleid=193378

2. Tse, I. (2011, February 11). 5 Ways Relationships Are Bad for Your Health. Retrieved March 9, 2015, from http://www.livescience.com/354695waysrelationshipsarebadforyour health.html

3. Tse, I. (2011, February 11). 5 Ways Relationships Are Bad for Your Health. Retrieved March 9, 2015, from http://www.livescience.com/354695waysrelationshipsarebadforyourhealth.html

4. Tse, I. (2011, February 11). 5 Ways Relationships Are Bad for Your Health. Retrieved February 24, 2015, from h ttp://www.livescience.com/354965waysrelationshipsarebadforyourhealth.html

5. Tse, I. (2011, February 11). 5 Ways Relationships Are Bad for Your Health. Retrieved March 3, 2015, from http://www.livescience.com/354695waysrelationshipsarebadforyourhealth.html

6. Umberson, D., & Montez, J. (2011, August 4). Social Relationships and Health: A Flashpoint for Health Policy. Retrieved January 1, 2015, from http://www.ncbi.nlm.nih.gov/pmc/ articles/PMC3150158/References

7. Umberson, D., & Montez, J. (2011, August 4). Social Relationships and Health: A Flashpoint for Health Policy. Retrieved January 4, 2015, from http://www.ncbi.nlm.nih.gov/pmc/ articles/PMC3150158/

8. Umberson, D., & Montez, J. (2011, August 4). Social Relationships and Health: A Flashpoint for Health Policy. Retrieved January 7, 2015, from http://www.ncbi.nlm.nih.gov/pmc/ articles/PMC3150158/

9. Umberson, D., & Montez, J. (2011, August 4). Social Relationships and Health: A Flashpoint for Health Policy. Retrieved January 9, 2015, from http://www.ncbi.nlm.nih.gov/pmc/ articles/PMC3150158/

10. Johnson, K. (2008). The Importance of Relationships. In T. Chobotar (Ed.), Creating Outstanding Relationships (Vol. 6, p. 10). Maitland, Florida: Florida Hospital Publishing.

11. Johnson, K. (2008). The Importance of Relationships. In T. Chobotar (Ed.), Creating Outstanding Relationships (Vol. 6, p. 10). Maitland, Florida: Florida Hospital Publishing.

12. Seven Psychological Sins [Motion picture on DVD]. (2013). United States: LifeHealth Network.

13. Seven Psychological Sins [Motion picture on DVD]. (2013). United States: LifeHealth Network.

14. Seven Psychological Sins [Motion picture on DVD]. (2013). United States: LifeHealth Network.

Habit #12 Thoughts

1. Goodwin, G. (2006). Depression and Associated Physical Diseases and Symptoms. Dialogues in Clinical Neuroscience. 259-265. Retrieved March 1, 2015, from Dialogues in Clinical Neuroscience.

2. Depression. Centers for Disease Control. (2013, October 4). Retrieved April 13, 2015, from http://www.cdc.gov/mentalhealth/basics/mentalillness/depression.htm

3. Stress Management. Mayo Clinic. (March 04, 2014). Retrieved March 6, 2015, from http://www.mayoclinic.org/healthylifestyle/stressmanagement/basics/stressbasics/hlv2 0049495

4. Causes and Effects of Stress: Family, Work, Health, and Other Stress Factors. WebMD. (n.d.).Retrieved from February 3, 2015, from http://www.webmd.com/balance/guide/causesofstress

Habit #13 Spirituality

1. Holt Lunstad, J., Steffen, P., Sandberg, J., & Jensen, B. (2011). Understanding the connection between spiritual wellbeing and physical health: An examination of ambulatory blood pressure, inflammation, blood lipids and fasting glucose. Journal of Behavioral Medicine, 477488. Retrieved from PubMed.gov.

2. Miller, L., Wickramaratne, P., Gameroff, M., Sage, M., Tenke, C., & Weissman, M. (2011). Religiosity and Major Depression in Adults at High Risk: A TenYear Prospective Study. American Journal of Psychiatry, 169(1), 8994. Retrieved November 14, 2014, from http://ajp.psychiatryonline.org/doi/ref/10.1176/appi.ajp.2011.10121823

Habit #14 Service

1. Sneed, R., & Cohen, S. (2013). A Prospective Study of Volunteerism and Hypertension Risk in Older Adults. National Institute of Health, 578586. Retrieved January 10, 2015, from National Institute of Health.

2. Sneed, R., & Cohen, S. (2013). A Prospective Study of Volunteerism and Hypertension Risk in Older Adults. National Institute of Health, 578586. Retrieved January 10, 2015, from National Institute of Health

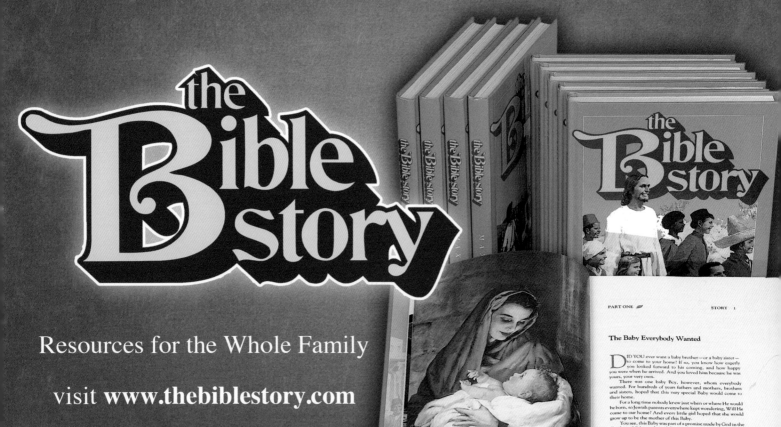
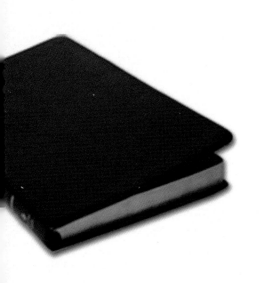
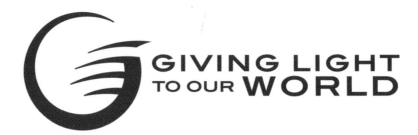